Practice Test #1

Practice Questions

1. Following a chest infection, a patient with type 1 diabetes reports fatigue and nausea. Assessment reveals a blood glucose level of 450 mg/dL. Which of the following pharmacologic interventions are priorities for patient care?
    a. Administer intravenous (IV) fluids at the prescribed rate to correct sodium levels.
    b. Administer intravenous (IV) fluids based on corrected sodium levels.
    c. Administer prescribed insulin via IV bolus, then continuous drip.
    d. B and C.

2. Which of the following are possible complications from diabetic ketoacidosis?
    a. Metabolic acidosis
    b. Hyperkalemia
    c. Metabolic alkalosis
    d. Hyponitremia

3. At discharge, the family of a patient who has had an episode of diabetes ketoacidosis wants to know how to care for their family member if they get sick at home. What should the nurse tell them? More than one answer may be correct.
    a. Continue to follow prescribed diabetic medications as usual and report a glucose reading of >300 mg/dL or urine ketones to the patient's physician.
    b. If the patient becomes nauseated, eat small meals and discontinue diabetic medications until nausea passes.
    c. If the patient has vomiting or persistent diarrhea, discontinue diabetic medications until vomiting stops.
    d. Test blood or glucose every 3 to 4 hours.

4. A nurse in the emergency department assesses a patient with a hand laceration and notices that the patient smells strongly of alcohol. The patient is diabetic, irritable, and pale and reports headache. The nurse is waiting for laboratory results. What serum glucose level might the nurse expect to find?
    a. 80 to 110 mg/dL
    b. <50 mg/dL
    c. 50 to 60 mg/dL
    d. >1000 mg/dL

5. An unconscious patient with hypoglycemia is being treated with IV glucose (50 mL of 50% dextrose IV bolus) to correct serum glucose levels of 40 mg/dL. Which of the following is a possible complication of administering hypertonic dextrose?
    a. Phlebitis
    b. Hypokalemia
    c. Myocardial infarction
    d. Cardiac arrest

6. A 27-year-old patient with rheumatoid arthritis is admitted with anemia. During administration of 200 mL packed red blood cells (PRBCs) over 1 hour, the patient becomes restless. Her pulse is bounding, and her blood pressure is elevated. The most likely explanation is:
    a. Hemolytic reaction to the transfusion
    b. The PRBCs are contaminated with gram-negative organisms
    c. The transfusion was administered too quickly
    d. Allergic response to the transfusion

7. Complications associated with long-term transfusions for sickle cell anemia patients include:
    a. Acute chest syndrome
    b. Stroke
    c. Alloimmunization
    d. Renal dysfunction

8. Which of the following laboratory results would the nurse expect to find with a patient who has heparin-induced thrombocytopenia (HIT)?
    a. 5 to 14 days following initiation of heparin therapy, platelet count drops 30% to 50% from the patient's baseline.
    b. 5 to 14 days following initiation of heparin therapy, platelet count increases 30% to 50% from the patient's baseline.
    c. Following initiation of heparin therapy, red blood cell count levels are increased.
    d. Following initiation of heparin therapy, red blood cell count levels are decreased.

9. A patient with rheumatoid arthritis and acute leukemia is admitted with a cough following a first cycle of chemotherapy. Assessment reveals hypotension, temperature of 38.4 degrees Celsius, and absolute neutrophil count of <500 cells/μL. The *MOST ESSENTIAL* nursing action is:
    a. Provide and encourage meticulous skin, peri-anal, and oral hygiene for the patient.
    b. Cleanse hands thoroughly before and after all direct patient contact. Ensure that staff caring for the patient have no signs and symptoms of infection.
    c. A and B
    d. Administer antipyretics.

10. What life-threatening reaction is associated with sickle cell anemia treatment agents?
    a. Myelosuppression
    b. Tinnitus
    c. Myopathy
    d. Hemorrhage

11. Minute ventilation (VE) is composed of:
    a. Alveolar ventilation (VA)
    b. Alveolar ventilation (VA) + physiologic dead space ventilation (VD)
    c. Tidal volume
    d. Tidal volume + respiratory rate

12. Which of the following *BEST* reflects the main purpose of the pulmonary system?
    a. To exchange oxygen and carbon dioxide in the atmosphere
    b. To exchange oxygen and carbon monoxide between the atmosphere and alveoli
    c. To exchange oxygen and carbon monoxide between the atmosphere and all body cells
    d. To exchange oxygen and carbon dioxide between the atmosphere and all body cells

13. Which of the following adventitious breath sounds are associated with fluid in the small airways?
    a. Crackles
    b. Wheezes
    c. Rhonchi
    d. Pleural friction rub

14. A patient with a history of pulmonary disease needs to be evaluated for hypoxemia. She asks the nurse what this will involve. Which of the following should the nurse tell the patient?
    a. A blood test will be taken and analyzed.
    b. A sensor will be placed on the patient's fingertip to measure levels of oxygen in her blood.
    c. The patient will be asked to blow into a machine that will measure tidal volume.
    d. The patient will be asked to exercise on a treadmill while attached to monitoring equipment. A blood sample will also be taken for testing.

15. A 59-year-old man with a history of chronic obstructive pulmonary disease is admitted with increasing breathlessness. On assessment he seems restless and confused. His pulse is rapid and bounding, and his blood pressure is elevated. Which of the following is most likely?
    a. Metabolic acidosis
    b. Respiratory acidosis
    c. Respiratory alkalosis
    d. Metabolic alkalosis

16. When the nurse is assessing a patient for respiratory disease, the nurse should *FIRST*:
    a. Ask the patient specific questions about activity and breathing based on their typical daily activities.
    b. Palpate the patient's chest.
    c. Check the patient's pulse rate.
    d. Request a sputum sample.

17. When the chest wall is palpated, what does a barrel chest typically indicate?
    a. Pneumothorax
    b. Emphysema
    c. Acute bronchitis
    d. Pulmonary embolism

18. A 28-year-old man is admitted with chest pain, tachycardia, and dyspnea. The patient's history reveals he was playing football when another player tackled him to the ground. Based on this information, what is the most likely diagnosis?
    a. Asthma
    b. Myocardial infarction
    c. Pneumothorax
    d. Pulmonary embolism

19. A patient with pneumothorax has a chest tube *in situ* to evacuate air. When monitoring the bottle, the nurse notices constant bubbling into the water. Which of the following should the nurse do *FIRST*?
    a. Check for a leak in the apparatus.
    b. Take a sample of the drainage fluid for laboratory analysis.
    c. Clamp the tube and disconnect the water seal drainage system.
    d. Suggest to the physician that a chest x-ray is required.

20. Symptoms of airflow obstruction and poor ventilation include:
    a. Nasal flaring
    b. Intercostal retractions
    c. Pursed lip breathing
    d. All of the above

21. Which of the following is an abnormal finding on inspection of an adult patient's chest?
    a. Respiratory rate of 12 to 20 breaths/minute
    b. Chest symmetry
    c. Quiet respirations
    d. Inspiration lasting twice as long as expiration

22. Atelectasis occurs in a 78-year-old postoperative patient. On physical examination, the nurse would *NOT* expect to find:
    a. Decreased respiratory rate and decreased pulse rate
    b. Absent or decreased tactile fremitus
    c. Breath sounds decreased or absent on the affected side
    d. Delayed chest expansion on the affected side

23. A 61-year-old woman with multiple sclerosis and a sacral pressure ulcer is being treated for pneumonia. During a dressing change, she becomes short of breath. On assessment, her blood pressure is low, pulse is rapid, and her skin is pale and moist. If these symptoms indicate acute respiratory failure, which of the following should the nurse do *FIRST*?
    a. Prepare intubation equipment.
    b. Increase the patient's IV infusion rate.
    c. Raise the bed to 30 degrees to maximize ventilation, and call the physician.
    d. Administer 40% oxygen via nasal cannula.

24. An underweight 67-year-old woman is admitted with an audible expiratory wheeze. She has a history of a productive cough for the previous 6 months. Laboratory findings confirm chronic bronchitis. The patient is widowed, lives on her own, and has smoked cigarettes for 40 years. What is the priority for discharge planning?
    a. Arrange for a dietician to develop a plan to help the patient regain muscle strength.
    b. Recommend physical therapy to promote strength training.
    c. Discuss a smoking cessation plan.
    d. Instruct the patient on the use of an inhaler.

25. The nurse is discharging a 24-year-old woman who presented with persistent coughing, wheezing, and shortness of breath on aerobic exercise. Her diagnosis was exercise-induced asthma (EIA). Which of the following is *MOST* important to educate the patient about controlling EIA?
    a. Switch to a nonaerobic form of exercise such as swimming.
    b. Suggest the patient take nonsteroidal anti-inflammatory drugs (NSAIDs) before exercise.
    c. Encourage the patient to take a bronchodilator 15 to 20 minutes before exercise.
    d. Avoid exercise.

26. The nurse is performing tracheotomy stoma care for a patient on mechanical ventilation who is being weaned from the tracheostomy tube. The patient's family asks what will happen when the patient's tube is removed. What should the nurse tell the family?
    a. When the patient is alert, the tube will be removed.
    b. When the patient is breathing independently, the tube will be removed.
    c. The respiratory therapist will monitor blood gas studies to determine when the tube should be removed.
    d. The respiratory therapist will make gradual changes to the tube size and cuff to ensure the patient can tolerate decannulation.

27. Following surgery to reduce a fractured neck of femur with internal fixation, a 78-year-old woman develops dyspnea and tachypnea. The respiratory therapist suspects pulmonary embolism and draws arterial blood for analysis. Which of the following tests would the nurse also expect?
    a. D-dimer assay
    b. Chest X-ray
    c. Pulmonary angiography
    d. All of the above

28. The respiratory generator is located in the:
    a. Chemoreceptors
    b. Cerebral cortex
    c. Medulla
    d. Diaphragm

29. A 37-year-old obese woman with a history of obstructive sleep apnea is being discharged. Which of the following best describes the *MAIN* priority for her home care?
    a. Medications to reduce residual daytime sleepiness
    b. Oxygen therapy via CPAP or BiPAP device
    c. Nocturnal oximetry monitoring
    d. Weight reduction program and oxygen therapy via CPAP or BiPAP device

30. The pericardium functions to:
    a. Encase the epicardial coronary arteries
    b. Attach the chordae tendineae to the ventricular chambers
    c. Protect the heart from friction
    d. Allow unidirectional blood flow

31. Coronary blood flow rate is approximately:
    a. 110 to 130 mL/min
    b. 90 to ≤110 mL/min
    c. 70 to ≤90 mL/min
    d. 50 to ≤70 mL/min

- 6 -

32. Coronary blood flow is reduced by:
    a. Bradycardia
    b. Hypertension
    c. Cardiac tamponade
    d. Tachycardia

33. The main function of parasympathetic stimulation is to:
    a. Release acetylcholine
    b. Increase sinoatrial (SA) node discharge
    c. Increase atrioventricular (AV) conduction time
    d. Release norepinephrine

34. In the cardiac conduction system, the left bundle branch system:
    a. Transmits impulse to the septum and left ventricle
    b. Conducts impulse to the bundle of His
    c. Delays impulse between atria and ventricles
    d. Depolarizes myocardium

35. On an electrocardiogram, a P wave represents:
    a. Atrial repolarization
    b. Ventricular polarization
    c. Ventricular repolarization
    d. Atrial depolarization

36. Cardiac index is based on:
    a. Cardiac output (CO)
    b. CO + ejection fraction (EF)
    c. Body surface area (BSA)
    d. Body mass index (BMI)

37. The automatic nervous system is comprised of which 2 elements:
    a. Venous system and cholinergic system
    b. Capillary system and venous system
    c. Adrenergic system and cholinergic system
    d. Adrenergic system and venous system

38. On auscultation of the heart, a high-pitched blowing murmur typically indicates:
    a. Heart failure
    b. Mitral insufficiency
    c. Mitral stenosis
    d. Arterial septal defect

39. A 53-year-old man with a history of recent myocardial infarction requires chest imaging. The nurse should anticipate:
    a. Cardiac catheterization and angiography
    b. Ultrafast electric beam computerized tomography (EBCT)
    c. Magnetic resonance imaging (MRI)
    d. Aortography

40. A 12-lead electrocardiogram (ECG) is administered to a 35-year-old man with acute chest pain, but his ECG complex is normal. In a normal ECG complex, the nurse should *NOT* see:
   a. ST segment following the QRS complex
   b. P wave that lasts <0.10 sec
   c. QRS complex with a duration of 0.06 to 0.01 sec
   d. P wave that lasts >0.10 sec

41. Lead II of a 12-lead ECG shows a rate of <50 beats/min, and normal RQRST complexes and intervals. The nurse should interpret this as an indication of:
   a. Sinus bradycardia
   b. Sinus pause
   c. Sinus arrhythmia
   d. Sinus rhythm

42. An electrocardiogram (ECG) on a 47-year-old man with a history of palpitations and blackouts shows irregularly irregular fibrillatory waves and a wide, complex tachycardia. The nurse should interpret this as:
   a. Atrial flutter
   b. Atrial fibrillation
   c. Ventricular fibrillation
   d. Ventricular tachycardia

43. On assessment, a 63-year-old man has cold, clammy skin, chest pain, and blood pressure of 85/60 mmHg. The problem underlying these findings is most likely:
   a. Dysrhythmias
   b. Increased cardiac output
   c. Decreased cardiac output
   d. Diaphoresis

44. A 69-year-old woman with angina complains of chest discomfort and shortness of breath. The nurse places the patient in a semi-Fowler position. This involves:
   a. Placing the patient in a supine position on a surface with a 45-degree incline. The patient's head is at the lower end and the knees are flexed over the upper end.
   b. Positioning the patient on the left side and chest, with the right knee and thigh drawn up, and the left arm along the back.
   c. Placing the patient in a supine position with hips and knees flexed and thighs abducted and externally rotated.
   d. Raising the head of the patient 12 to 18 inches above the surface level and elevating the patient's knees.

45. On discharging a male patient with stable angina, the nurse should ensure that the patient is educated about his medications. Which of the following is *NOT* recommended for the pharmacologic treatment of angina?
   a. Diuretics
   b. Nitroglycerin
   c. Calcium antagonists
   d. Statins

46. Following cardiac revascularization via percutaneous transluminal coronary angioplasty (PTCA), a 190-kg male patient is receiving weight-based unfractionated heparin (UFH) to prevent thrombus formation. The nurse monitors the latest activated partial thrombin time (APTT) results. The APTT goal should be:
    a. 30 to 40 seconds
    b. 1.5 to 2 times the normal value
    c. 0.5 to 1.5 times the normal value
    d. 60 to 70 seconds

47. A patient with chest pain is suspected of having experienced a myocardial infarction. Electrocardiogram shows changes on leads V1-V2, which suggests that the septal wall was the area of infarct. If so, which artery is involved?
    a. Posterior descending artery
    b. Right coronary artery
    c. Left circumflex artery
    d. Left anterior descending artery

48. Immediately following craniotomy for closed head trauma, a 29-year-old man sustains a ST-segment elevation myocardial infarction (STEMI). Which of the following interventions is contraindicated?
    a. Fibrinolysis
    b. Percutaneous coronary intervention
    c. Thrombolysis
    d. Intra-aortic balloon pump

49. Following a diagnosis of myocarditis, a 58-year-old male patient has a permanent pacemaker inserted. The nurse should ensure the patient understands about the need to:
    a. Avoid hiccups
    b. Check his pulse daily at home
    c. Make sure his pacemaker is charged
    d. Prevent pacemaker syndrome

50. A 72-year-old woman is admitted following a fall at home. Her pulse is 52 bpm, and laboratory results show a serum potassium level of 5.8 mEq/L. The physician diagnoses sick sinus syndrome. Which of the following is the most likely management?
    a. Beta-blockers
    b. Stent
    c. Pacemaker implantation
    d. Statin therapy

51. The nurse assesses a 63-year-old woman postoperatively following coronary artery bypass grafting. The patient is hypotensive and has weak peripheral pulses and an increased respiratory rate; laboratory results reveal increased blood urea nitrogen. The physician thinks the patient may be suffering from acute cardiac tamponade. Which of the following diagnostic procedures will the physician request?
    a. Cardiac catheterization
    b. Transesophageal echocardiogram
    c. Holter monitor
    d. Echocardiography

52. The nurse needs to help a patient calculate body mass index as part of the patient's discharge plan. Which of the following is the correct calculation?
    a. BMI = Weight (lb) / (Height (in) x Height (in))
    b. BMI = Weight (kg) / (Height (m) x Height (m)) x 703
    c. BMI = Weight (lb) / (Height (in) x Height (in)) x 703
    d. BMI = Weight (kg) / (Height (m)

53. The nurse managing a patient with ischemic cardiomyopathy is titrating an IV dose of norepinephrine bitartrate. The order is written to start at 8 mcg/min and titrate to systolic blood pressure greater than 90 mmHg. Which of the following should the nurse do?
    a. Double-check the dose limit with the physician
    b. Assess the patient's peripheral circulation before titrating
    c. Check the patient's hemodynamic parameters with noninvasive blood-pressure monitoring
    d. Assess the patient's serum potassium before titrating

54. A patient with syncope is diagnosed with a conduction defect, and a transcutaneous pacemaker is ordered. The purpose of this is to:
    a. Increase blood flow through the arteries
    b. Provide an extrinsic electrical impulse so that depolarization and subsequent contraction can occur
    c. Transmit radiofrequency energy to heart muscle
    d. Increase the pumping motion of the heart

55. Following pacemaker insertion, a 67-year-old woman reports sharp, stabbing chest pain. She feels anxious and is trying to get out of bed. On assessment, the patient has pulsus paradoxus and dyspnea. Which of the following should the nurse do *IMMEDIATELY*?
    a. Lay the patient flat and initiate cardiopulmonary resuscitation
    b. Place the patient in a high Fowler position and secure the airway
    c. Place the patient in the Trendelenburg position and notify the physician
    d. Elevate the head of the patient's bed and notify the physician

56. The nurse monitoring a 64-year-old male patient 6 hours after coronary artery bypass grafting notes that his blood pressure is 180/95 mmHg. Which pharmacologic agent would *NOT* be prescribed?
    a. Diuretics
    b. Vasodilators
    c. Calcium channel blockers
    d. Adrenergic inhibitors

57. The family of a patient who has had surgery to repair an abdominal aortic aneurysm asks the nurse to explain the condition to them. The nurse should tell the family that an abdominal aortic aneurysm is:
    a. A dilatation of the arterial wall of the aorta of at least 50%
    b. A congenital deformity of the aorta that creates a narrowing of the lumen and reduces blood flow
    c. Atherosclerosis of the medial wall of the ascending or descending aorta
    d. Abnormal narrowing of the aortic valve

58. A 65-year-old woman is admitted with chest pain and a preliminary diagnosis of aortic dissection. The signs and symptoms associated with aortic dissection can be differentiated from those associated with myocardial infarction by which of the following?
    a. Cramping, aching pain with exertion
    b. Instantaneous onset of severe pain and absence of pulses
    c. Chest pain accompanied by tachycardia
    d. Cramping, aching pain on rest

59. A 58-year-old male patient with diabetes is admitted with a history of weakness in his legs during activity. On examination, his blood pressure is 158/98 mmHg; his dorsalis pedalis is weak; and the skin on his feet is reddened. The most likely treatment for this patient is:
    a. Antihypertensive medications and exercise therapy
    b. Blood tests for serum glucose
    c. Antihypertensive medications and rest
    d. Exercise therapy and serum glucose monitoring

60. The nurse is monitoring an obese 56-year-old female patient following a right knee replacement. The patient becomes breathless; on examination, her pulse is rapid, she is sweating, and her right leg is warm to the touch, with prominent veins. The nurse's primary concern for the patient is:
    a. Cardiogenic shock
    b. Myocardial infarction
    c. Aortic disruption
    d. Pulmonary embolism

61. Following the onset of acute myocardial infarction, a 70-year-old male patient has a blood pressure of 75/48 mmHg and oliguria. The most appropriate pharmacologic intervention to manage cardiogenic shock in this case would be:
    a. IV bolus administration of 3% ephedrine 5 mg at 15 minute intervals
    b. IV administration of dopamine 3 mcg/kg/minute via infusion pump
    c. IV bolus administration of 1:10,000 adrenaline 1 mL until effective
    d. IV administration of potassium chloride

62. Following reperfusion after an episode of cardiogenic shock, the nurse is reviewing laboratory results and notices that blood urea nitrogen (BUN) levels for the patient are elevated. Normal values for BUN are:
    a. 10 to 20 mg/dL
    b. 10:1 to 20:1
    c. 40 to 60 mg/dL
    d. 5 to 10 mg/dL

63. A 76-year-old female patient with coronary artery disease has poorly controlled weight and reports tiredness and difficulty sleeping. On examination, the patient's blood pressure is 85/58 mm/Hg; pulse is 126/min; and she has pitting edema. The nurse anticipates the physician will order:
    a. 0.5% IV Ringer solution
    b. Oral fludrocortisones 0.1 mg/day
    c. IV furosemide 5 mg/hour
    d. IV bolus 0.25 mg/kg diltiazem

64. The nurse is monitoring a 69-year-old male patient who is being treated for Cushing syndrome. He complains of headache and nausea. On assessment, his blood pressure is 210/126 mmHg. Which of the following interventions should the nurse anticipate?
    a. Administration of nitroprusside and transfer to ICU
    b. Administration of adrenaline and transfer to ICU
    c. Administration of dextran 70 and close monitoring
    d. Administration of heparin and transfer to ICU

65. Which of the following is *NOT* an indication of complications from hypertensive crisis?
    a. Dysrhythmia
    b. Lowered intracranial pressure
    c. Raised intracranial pressure
    d. Elevated blood pressure

66. In mitral regurgitation, blood is partially regurgitated into the:
    a. Right atrium
    b. Right ventricle
    c. Left atrium
    d. Left ventricle

67. On assessing a 70-year-old woman who has been admitted with fatigue, palpitations, and dyspnea on exertion, the nurse learns that the patient had rheumatic fever as a child. Rheumatic fever is a risk factor for which of the following?
    a. Mitral valve prolapse
    b. Mitral stenosis
    c. Aortic coarctation
    d. Aortic dissection

68. A 62-year-old woman has been diagnosed with new-onset atrial fibrillation and is scheduled for transthoracic cardioversion. Which of the following is a complication arising from transthoracic cardioversion?
    a. Heartburn
    b. Ventricular fibrillation
    c. Myocardial infarction
    d. Hypokalemia

69. A 68-year-old male patient with supraventricular tachycardia of recent onset is scheduled for pharmacologic cardioversion. Which of the following is *NOT* a contraindication for pharmacologic cardioversion?
    a. Atrial fibrillation
    b. Hemodynamic instability
    c. Marked bradycardia
    d. Hypokalemia

70. A 72-year-old patient who has been admitted for anti-arrhythmic therapy to treat paroxysmal atrial tachycardia suddenly becomes pale. On examination, the nurse observes that the patient is pulseless. Which of the following actions should the nurse take *FIRST*?
    a. Administer IV epinephrine
    b. Begin cardiopulmonary resuscitation
    c. Alert the response team and begin basic life-support protocols
    d. Apply electric shock

71. The glomerular filtration rate (GFR) is the:
    a. Serum sodium concentration level
    b. Sodium reabsorption rate
    c. Volume of plasma cleared of a given substance per minute
    d. Volume of urine cleared of a given substance per minute

72. The products of excretion measured for interpretation of renal function are:
    a. BUN and creatinine
    b. BUN and sodium
    c. Creatinine and sodium
    d. BUN and potassium

73. During a shift change, the nurse monitoring a 67-year-old female patient who is being treated for pericarditis notes that the patient's urine output for the previous 4 hours decreased to <30 mL/hr. Nursing intervention should include:
    a. Increasing fluid and sodium intake and alerting nephrologist
    b. Increasing fluid intake, monitoring changes in urea and electrolytes, and alerting nephrologist
    c. Increasing sodium intake, monitoring changes in urea and electrolytes, and alerting nephrologist
    d. Reducing fluid intake, monitoring changes in urea and electrolytes, and alerting nephrologist

74. A 45-year-old male patient with a history of chronic pyelonephritis and end-stage renal disease (ESRD) is assessed by the nurse. Which of the following is the leading cause of ESRD?
    a. Diabetes mellitus
    b. Pyelonephritis
    c. Diabetic nephropathy
    d. Diabetic insipidus

75. Nursing assessment of a 45-year-old woman reporting epigastric pain reveals that she has abdominal tenderness, hyperactive bowel sounds, nausea and vomiting, and weight loss. The physician orders an upper GI series to rule out which of the following?
    a. Crohn's disease
    b. Diverticulitis
    c. Duodenal ulcer
    d. Ulcerative colitis

76. A 48-year-old man with cirrhosis is hospitalized for treatment of spontaneous bacterial peritonitis. During the morning shift, he suddenly vomits projectile coffee ground–like material; on examination, his blood pressure is low and he has a tachycardia. Which of the following is the most likely explanation for these signs and symptoms?
    a. Pancreatitis
    b. Esophageal varices
    c. Esophagitis
    d. Colitis

77. Laboratory results for a 56-year-old female patient with abdominal pain show decreased hemoglobin, hematocrit, potassium, and albumin levels; fecal occult blood; and a raised white blood cell count. On review of the abdominal X-ray, the physician diagnoses Crohn's disease. Which of the following did the physician most likely see on the X-ray?
    a. Irregular widening of distal ileum
    b. Narrowed loops of bowel
    c. Dilated loops of bowel
    d. Irregular narrowing of distal ileum

78. The nurse monitoring a patient with acute pancreatitis being managed by total parenteral nutrition (TPN) observes that he has an irregular pulse. The patient's laboratory results show serum potassium of 2.5 mEq/L and markedly high blood glucose levels. Which of the following actions should the nurse take?
    a. Adjust the insulin dose and electrolytes in the TPN solution
    b. Administer water as 5% dextrose via a peripheral vein
    c. Adjust the dextrose solution from 5% to 25% in the TPN solution
    d. Adjust the dextrose solution to 50% in the TPN solution

79. The main function of the blood-brain barrier is to regulate:
    a. Influences on the coordination of voluntary motion
    b. Emotional behavioral responses
    c. Collateral circulation
    d. Movement of certain substances from blood into brain tissue

80. The primary neurotransmitter of the peripheral nervous system is:
    a. Norepinephrine
    b. Acetylcholine
    c. Dopamine
    d. Glutamate

81. A 37-year-old female patient has a GCS score of 6. The GCS assesses:
    a. Motor function
    b. Pathologic reflexes
    c. Level of consciousness
    d. Peripheral nerve lesions

82. A 52-year-old woman is admitted with severe headache, nausea, and dizziness. She cannot flex her neck, and a CT scan reveals an intracranial aneurysm. The patient's family asks the nurse what will happen next. Which of the following is most likely?
    a. Craniotomy
    b. Embolization
    c. Surgical repair
    d. Proton beam

83. A 57-year-old man is admitted with left-sided ischemic stroke and is considered a good candidate for tissue plasminogen activator (t-PA), which is started via IV. At shift change, the nurse caring for this patient observes that his blood pressure is 185/100 mmHg, and his pupils are poorly reactive. For which of the following events is this patient at risk?
    a. Intracranial aneurysm
    b. Hemorrhagic stroke
    c. Increased intracranial pressure
    d. Seizure

84. A 35-year-old human immunodeficiency virus (HIV)–positive man is admitted for investigation of recurrent epistaxis. On assessment, the patient is pale, has purpura, and laboratory tests show a platelet count of 45,000/mm³ and hemoglobin level of 10 g/dL. Which is the following is a common hematological complication of HIV?
    a. Thrombocytopenia
    b. Pneumonia
    c. Myelopathy
    d. Encephalopathy

85. A 42-year-old primigravida patient with diabetes is being treated for placental abruption. On assessment, the nurse notes petechiae and blood oozing from the patient's IV line. The patient's blood pressure is 90/55 mmHg, and her temperature is 102°F. Following measures to treat the underlying causes of disseminated intravascular coagulation (DIC), which of the following laboratory results provides evidence of patient improvement?
    a. Hemoglobin (HGB) level higher than 7 g/dL
    b. Platelet count higher than 50,000/mm3
    c. Hematocrit (HCT) of 21%
    d. Raised erythrocyte sedimentation rate (ESR)

86. Which of the following physical examination/laboratory results is NOT a manifestation of systemic inflammatory response syndrome (SIRS)?
    a. Temperature >100.4°F (38°C)
    b. Heart rate >90 bpm
    c. White blood count >4000/mm3 or <12,000/mm3
    d. PaCO2 of <32 mmHg

87. A 10-year-old girl is receiving treatment for her second bee sting of the summer. She has facial edema, tachycardia, and is wheezing when suddenly she stops breathing and loses consciousness. Which of the following drugs should the nurse prepare to treat the patient's hypersensitivity?
    a. Epinephrine 0.5 mL of 1:1000 IV
    b. Epinephrine 0.2 mL of 1:1000 IV
    c. Epinephrine 0.5 mL of 1:10000 IV
    d. Epinephrine 0.2 mL of 1:10000 IV

88. Following abdominal surgery, a patient becomes flushed and distressed. On assessment, the nurse notes that the patient's temperature is 102°F, heart rate is 102/bpm, and urinary output for the last two hours has been reduced, at 25 mL/hour. The nurse should consider these to be clinical manifestations of which of the following conditions?
   a. Wound dehiscence
   b. Sepsis
   c. Anaphylactic shock
   d. Type I hypersensitivity

89. Survival for patients diagnosed with septic shock is improved by using early goal-directed therapy. Which of the following therapies are *NOT* likely in treating septic shock?
   a. Antimicrobials
   b. Vasopressors
   c. Corticosteroids
   d. Diuretics

90. The nurse is catheterizing a 47-year-old female patient prior to surgery and at the end of the procedure lifts the drainage bag above the patient's body, putting the patient at risk for which of the following events?
   a. Infection
   b. Incontinence
   c. Urinary retention
   d. Urethral injury

91. Which of the following is the leading cause of death in ICUs?
   a. Sepsis
   b. Systemic inflammatory response syndrome (SIRS)
   c. Shock
   d. Cardiac arrest

92. Following 5 days in the ICU, a 24-year-old female patient is transferred to progressive care. After the first night, she reports not sleeping and becomes increasingly anxious. Which of the following approaches is acceptable for care of this patient?
   a. Establish a quiet environment
   b. Work with the patient to restore a normal sleeping pattern
   c. Provide sleep medication
   d. All of the above

93. A 58-year-old male patient shows signs of pain following abdominal surgery but refuses opioids based on a fear of addiction. Which of the following explanations should the nurse use to reassure the patient about opioids?
   a. The patient is entitled to refuse pain medications
   b. Opioids have a less than 1% addiction rate
   c. Admire the patient's stoicism
   d. Acknowledge opioid addiction potential and offer an alternative medication

94. A 47-year-old male patient is admitted for investigation of abdominal pain. Twenty-four hours after admission, he becomes restless and disoriented. His pulse is 110/bpm; he is sweating and develops tremors. Review of his chart reveals an elevated blood alcohol level on admission. Which of the following conditions is caused by withdrawal of alcohol?
  a. Anxiety
  b. Depression
  c. Delirium
  d. Psychosis

95. A 78-year-old female patient with dementia is admitted for emergency surgery for a fracture neck of femur. The patient is anxious and is unable to sleep. Which of the following medications might the physician order to help with anxiety and insomnia?
  a. Benzodiazepines
  b. Antipsychotics
  c. Lithium
  d. Neuroleptics

96. A 28-year-old male patient is being treated for acute pancreatitis when he becomes delirious, agitated, and abusive. He tries to get out of bed and pulls out his IV; consequently, restraints are ordered to protect the patient and staff. Which of the following nursing actions would be ethically inappropriate?
  a. Apply the restraints before the patient causes more harm
  b. Seek informed consent from the patient or his family before applying restraints
  c. Discuss alternative treatments with the patient and his family
  d. Determine whether the patient has decision-making capacity

97. A family-centered approach to patient care recognizes that families:
  a. May be harmful to a patient's full recovery
  b. Should be allowed to visit the patient at any time
  c. Are team members in the patient's healing process
  d. Should be included in all decisions about patient care

98. A 48-year-old female patient has been admitted for investigation of impaired vision, fatigue, muscle weakness, and poor coordination. A lumbar puncture is scheduled, prior to which the patient becomes upset and reports abdominal pain. The physician insists on continuing with the lumbar puncture. In the best interests of the patient, the nurse should:
  a. Reassure the patient that the procedure will be over soon
  b. Suggest rescheduling when the patient's abdominal pain has been investigated and stabilized
  c. Continue preparing the patient for the lumbar puncture
  d. Recommend pain relief and continue with the procedure

99. Which of the following statements illustrates that a nurse is being the patient's advocate?
  a. I was cold and the nurse brought me a blanket
  b. The nurse took the tape off my mother's IV even though it was tearing her skin
  c. The nurse didn't have an answer to my question but took the time to research it
  d. When the nurses say they will check back, they do

100. Which of the following patient statements *LEAST* reflects caring practice in progressive care nursing? The nurse:
    a. Was interested in me as a person
    b. Took a long time to respond to my request
    c. Put my mind at ease
    d. Appeared to like their job

101. A patient with a history of psychosis is 48 hours postoperative following an appendectomy. He becomes agitated, delusional, verbally abusive, and he hits a nurse who approaches him. Which of the following is the *FIRST* responsive action the nurse's colleague should take?
    a. Follow facility protocols for contacting facility security
    b. Communicate the risk of assault to other staff
    c. Request a psychiatric consult for the patient
    d. Administer first aid to the assault victim and assaultive patient, as appropriate

102. A 38-year-old woman is recovering from abdominal surgery. She has a wound drain and an IV line. Her 7-year-old son has not been sleeping and wants to visit his mother. Which of the following actions could the nurse take to demonstrate caring practices?
    a. Take the boy immediately to see his mother
    b. Explain to the boy what equipment he will see and what to expect when he sees his mother
    c. Explain that it will be best to wait until the patient's wound drain has been removed
    d. Explain that the boy will be able to see his mother in a few days

103. At the end of a shift, a 79-year-old female patient being treated for end-stage renal disease calls for a nurse. A nurse going off duty responds on her way out of the unit and finds that the patient is cold. Which of the following responses BEST indicates caring practice? The nurse:
    a. Tells the patient that she will get another nurse to find a blanket
    b. Finds an additional blanket and tucks in the patient
    c. Turns up the thermostat
    d. the patient call again for the nurse on this shift

104. A nurse is monitoring a patient just before a shift change and notices that the patient's peripheral IV has stopped. On inspection, there is swelling and tenderness at the venipuncture site, and it appears as though the IV has infiltrated. The patient's notes reveal this is the third infiltration in 24 hours. Which of the following actions by the nurse is an example of an inquiry-based approach?
    a. Stop the infusion and remove the device
    b. Identify if there is an underlying cause for infiltration
    c. Raise the patient's limb
    d. Change the IV tubing

105. The father of a 7-year-old girl who is being treated for acute lymphoblastic leukemia wishes to spend the night with his daughter. Although this is contrary to visiting policy, the child pleads with the nurse to allow her father to stay. Which of the following actions by the nurse is an example of an inquiry-based approach?
    a. Reassure the father that his daughter is well taken care of and suggest that he return early in the morning
    b. Allow the father to stay and evaluate the girl's response
    c. Suggest the father stays in the room with his daughter
    d. Recommend local motels

106. A 37-year-old male patient is admitted with upper epigastric pain, and a medical student has been detailed to insert a nasogastric tube under nursing supervision. The student instills X mL of viscous lidocaine 2% down the patient's nostril but does not ask the patient to sniff and swallow. Two attempts at intubation fail, and the patient shows signs of distress. Which of the following actions by the nurse is an example of an inquiry-based approach?
   a. Apologize to the patient
   b. Stop the procedure and take over the intubation
   c. Suggest an alternative anesthetic technique such as nebulization of lidocaine 1% or 4% through a face mask
   d. Ask the medical student to begin again

107. Following treatment for a chest infection, the nurse is arranging discharge for a patient with newly diagnosed type 1 diabetes who mentions that he struggles to understand how a low-fat diet helps his diabetes. Which of the following collaborating professionals should the nurse involve in this patient's care?
   a. Discharge planner
   b. Diabetic educator
   c. Consulting physician
   d. Endocrinologist

108. An 86-year-old man is admitted with pneumonia. He requires 100% O_2 via a nonbreather mask to maintain SpO_2 >90%. Which of the following collaborating professionals should the nurse involve in this patient's care?
   a. Physical therapist and respiratory therapist
   b. Cardiovascular technologist and physical therapist
   c. Pulmonary technician and cardiovascular technologist
   d. Respiratory therapist and pulmonary technician

109. A 27-year-old patient with diabetes and rheumatoid arthritis (RA) is admitted for treatment of anemia via administration of 200 mL packed red blood cells (PRBCs) over 1 hour. To promote collaboration, which of the following team members should be informed of this patient's admission?
   a. Rheumatologist
   b. Hematologist
   c. Endocrinologist
   d. Immunologist

110. A patient is being transitioned from medications via IV fluids to oral medications. In order to facilitate patient learning, which of the following actions is BEST for the nurse to take?
   a. Explain the purpose of each medication to the patient
   b. Ensure that the patient takes his medication at the appropriate time
   c. Ensure that that patient takes the appropriate medication dose
   d. Describe the side effects of the new medications

111. A 70-year-old Hispanic patient with a history of pulmonary disease needs to be evaluated for hypoxemia. Her family speaks very little English. Which of the following actions can the nurse take to help the family understand what hypoxemia evaluation will entail?
    a. Explain in English using short sentences and simple words
    b. Request an interpreter
    c. Show the patient and her family a picture of a treadmill and write out simple instructions
    d. Assume that the pulmonary technician will explain the evaluation procedure

112. A 48-year-old man who was admitted with chest pain, tachycardia, and dyspnea is treated for pneumothorax. He has a history of asthma. A newly qualified nurse is monitoring the patient and finds his blood pressure is 70/55 mmHg. The patient reports chest pain and trouble breathing. The nurse consults with a more experienced nurse colleague who recognizes the likelihood of a tension pneumothorax. Which of the following actions should the experienced nurse take to facilitate learning for the newly qualified nurse?
    a. Explain how to perform an emergency needle thoracostomy
    b. Call the physician and set out equipment for an emergency needle thoracostomy
    c. Ask the newly qualified nurse to secure the patient's airway
    d. Secure and maintain the patient's airway, then ask the newly qualified nurse to call the physician and set out equipment for an emergency needle thoracostomy

113. A 10-year-old Native American boy is admitted for treatment of status asthmaticus. When stable, the patient's grandmother visits and brings him licorice tea, a common herbal remedy in the Native American community. The nurse caring for the patient is anxious that the boy's family may not follow his medication regimen at home. Which of the following responses by the nurse respects the family's culture and maintains the patient's best interest?
    a. Ask the patient's grandmother to explain the benefits of licorice, and educate the patient's grandmother about the need to maintain the patient's medication regimen
    b. Explain to the patient's grandmother that licorice may not be helpful to the patient
    c. Ask the patient's grandmother to stop giving the patient licorice tea
    d. Tell the patient's grandmother about the correct use of inhalers

114. A 57-year-old Latino male patient with dyspnea and chest pain is being assessed by the nurse. The patient speaks little English, and the nurse speaks little Spanish. Which of the following actions by the nurse appropriately incorporates cultural differences into patient care?
    a. The nurse asks the patient's family for additional information
    b. The nurse uses a telephone interpreter
    c. The nurse attempts to speak Spanish to the patient
    d. The nurse checks the patient's vital signs and reviews his test results without speaking

115. A 62-year-old African American male patient is being monitored following treatment for myocardial infarction. The nurse assigned to his care cannot pronounce his name. Which of the following actions by the nurse respects the patient's identity?
    a. Use a term of endearment when addressing the patient, such as "dear"
    b. Ask the patient how he would like to be addressed
    c. Avoid using the patient's name
    d. Ask the patient to write his name

116. A busy progressive care unit often has staffing problems. Which of the following approaches effectively supports systems thinking?
    a. Ensure there are last-minute incentives for staff to meet immediate patient-care needs
    b. Set up an evaluation to identify the reason for scheduling problems in the unit
    c. Require nurses to schedule early
    d. Penalize nurses for scheduling at the last minute

117. A 55-year-old male patient has had a pacemaker fitted for treatment of a conduction defect and is being discharged. A systems thinking approach to discharge will ensure which of the following occurrences?
    a. The patient will have all of his medications
    b. The patient's wound will be clean and dry
    c. Discharge has been planned in collaboration with the cardiologist, physical therapist, and pharmacist
    d. Discharge has been planned with the strengths and needs of the patient in mind

118. A 61-year-old woman with multiple sclerosis and a sacral pressure ulcer is to be discharged following treatment for pneumonia. She lives alone. Which of the following strategies is a systems thinking approach to the patient's discharge?
    a. Educate the patient about respiratory and skin care
    b. Arrange for a physical therapist to consult with the patient
    c. Coordinate home care for the patient with the discharge planner
    d. Arrange for a home nursing service to monitor the patient's pressure ulcers

119. A patient arrives at the emergency department complaining of mid-sternal chest pain. Which of the following nursing action should take priority?
    a. A complete history with emphasis on preceding events.
    b. An electrocardiogram.
    c. Careful assessment of vital signs.
    d. Chest exam with auscultation.

120. A nurse is caring for an elderly Vietnamese patient in the terminal stages of lung cancer. Many family members are in the room around the clock performing unusual rituals and bringing ethnic foods. Which of the following actions should the nurse take?
    a. Restrict visiting hours and ask the family to limit visitors to two at a time.
    b. Notify visitors with a sign on the door that the patient is limited to clear fluids only with no solid food allowed.
    c. If possible, keep the other bed in the room unassigned to provide privacy and comfort to the family.
    d. Contact the physician to report the unusual rituals and activities.

121. A patient on the cardiac telemetry unit unexpectedly goes into ventricular fibrillation. The advanced cardiac life support team prepares to defibrillate. Which of the following choices indicates the correct placement of the conductive gel pads?
    a. The left clavicle and right lower sternum.
    b. Right of midline below the bottom rib and the left shoulder.
    c. The upper and lower halves of the sternum.
    d. The right side of the sternum just below the clavicle and left of the precordium.

122. A nurse cares for a patient who has a nasogastric tube attached to low suction because of a suspected bowel obstruction. Which of the following arterial blood gas results might be expected in this patient?
    a. pH 7.52, PCO2 54 mm Hg.
    b. pH 7.42, PCO2 40 mm Hg.
    c. pH 7.25, PCO2 25 mm Hg.
    d. pH 7.38, PCO2 36 mm Hg.

123. A patient is admitted to the hospital for routine elective surgery. Included in the list of current medications is Coumadin (warfarin) at a high dose. Concerned about the possible effects of the drug, particularly in a patient scheduled for surgery, the nurse anticipates which of the following actions?
    a. Draw a blood sample for prothrombin (PT) and international normalized ratio (INR) level.
    b. Administer vitamin K.
    c. Draw a blood sample for type and crossmatch and request blood from the blood bank.
    d. Cancel the surgery after the patient reports stopping the Coumadin one week previously.

124. The follow lab results are received for a patient. Which of the following results are abnormal? Note: More than one answer may be correct.
    a. Hemoglobin 10.4 g/dL.
    b. Total cholesterol 340 mg/dL.
    c. Total serum protein 7.0 g/dL.
    d. Glycosylated hemoglobin A1C 5.4%.

125. A patient is admitted to the hospital with a diagnosis of primary hyperparathyroidism. A nurse checking the patient's lab results would expect which of the following changes in laboratory findings?
    a. Elevated serum calcium.
    b. Low serum parathyroid hormone (PTH).
    c. Elevated serum vitamin D.
    d. Low urine calcium.

Answers and Explanations

1. D: IV fluids are administered for dehydration based on *corrected* sodium levels (protocols usually start with 0.9% normal saline [NS and progress to 0.45% NS and dextrose 5% in water per lab values). Prescribed insulin is administered until blood glucose level is normalized and maintained, taking care to monitor insulin levels.

2. A: Metabolic acidosis is caused by ketosis resulting from insulin deficiency and stress hormone excess. Hyperkalemia is caused by higher than normal levels of potassium, usually through impaired renal function. Hyponatremia is a low level of nitrogen in the blood associated with protein malnutrition or overhydration. Metabolic alkalosis is an acid-base imbalance, like metabolic acidosis, but is caused by an increase in serum bicarbonate (HCO_3^-) concentration.

3. A and D: The nurse should inform the patient and his family to follow "Sick Day Rules." If the patient is nauseous, he should eat frequent small meals of soft foods while continuing prescribed diabetic medications and if experiencing vomiting or diarrhea, increase caloric intake through liquids every 30 to 60 minutes. If nausea or vomiting persists, the patient should consult his physician.

4. B: Excessive alcohol intake is a risk factor for hypoglycemia because alcohol inhibits gluconeogenesis. Although the level of glucose that produces hypoglycemia varies from person to person—mild hypoglycemia may range from 60 to 70 mg/dL to severe hypoglycemia with very low levels of glucose (e.g., below 40 mg/dL)—hypoglycemia is generally described as a decrease in serum glucose at or below 50 mg/dL. A goal of patient care is to elevate and maintain serum glucose at 80 to 110 mg/dL. A serum glucose level of >1000 mg/dL is associated with hyperglycemic, hyperosmolar nonketotic syndrome (HHNS).

5. A: Hypoglycemia resulting from insulin excess or other causes in adults and children is typically treated with 20 to 50 mL of 50% dextrose injection administered slowly (eg, 3 mL/minute) IV. Hypertonic dextrose commonly causes phlebitis if a peripheral vein is used and should therefore be administered slowly.

6. C: Circulatory overload can happen any time during a transfusion and is likely when it is administered too quickly. It causes hypertension, bounding pulse, and restlessness. Treatment involves slowing the transfusion and monitoring the patient's progress. Hemolytic, bacterial, and allergic reactions typically occur soon after transfusion is initiated; hemolytic and bacterial reactions are accompanied by tachycardia, and allergic reaction is accompanied by hypotension.

7. C: Alloimmunization occurs when the patient develops antibodies against a range of antigens following repeated blood product transfusions. The transfused cells are destroyed and the transfusion fails to correct the patient's blood counts. A, B, and D are all complications of sickle cell anemia.

8. A: Although HIT is rare, it is triggered by the immune system 5 to 14 days following initiation of heparin therapy and causes a low platelet count. A decrease in platelet count that occurs before 5 days following heparin therapy is typically a transient condition called nonautoimmune heparin-associated thrombocytopenia. Complications include deep venous thrombosis.

9. C: Although anti-pyretics may be ordered by the physician, they may mask fever and should not be initiated by the nurse. Assessment and history suggest neutropenia and the patient is at risk of infection and septic shock.

10. A: Hemorrhage is associated with thrombolytics and anti-platelet agents; myopathy and tinnitus are associated with anti-fibrinolytics; and myelosuppression is associated with hydroxyurea.

11. B: Alveolar ventilation is one component of minute ventilation, which comprise of alveolar ventilation and physiologic dead space ventilation (VE = VD+ VA). Minute ventilation is equal to exhaled tidal volume (VT) multiplied by respiratory rate (RR).

12. D: The pulmonary system exchanges oxygen and carbon dioxide between the atmosphere and alveoli, between alveoli and pulmonary capillary blood, and between systemic capillary blood and blood cells. Carbon monoxide is not involved in healthy gas exchange.

13. A: Crackles (or rales) are caused by fluid in the small airways or atelectasis. Wheezes (B) are caused by air moving through airways narrowed by constriction or obstruction. Rhonchi (C) is another term for wheezes. Pleural friction rub (D) is a grating or creaking sound that occurs when inflamed pleural surfaces rub together during respiration.

14. D: Exercise testing is used to evaluate hypoxemia, using a treadmill or other equipment tailored to patient ability. Arterial blood gases and/or SpO_2 confirm or rule out oxygen desaturation during exercise. Although pulse oximetry provides a continuous measure of arterial oxyhemoglobin, arterial blood is also required to evaluate desaturation on exertion.

15. B: Respiratory acidosis is a pH imbalance that results from alveolar hypoventilation and an accumulation of carbon dioxide. Chronic respiratory acidosis is seen in patients with chronic pulmonary disease. Metabolic acidosis (A) is caused by ketosis resulting from insulin deficiency and stress hormone excess. Respiratory alkalosis (C) is a pH imbalance that results from the excessive loss of carbon dioxide through hyperventilation. Metabolic alkalosis (D) is caused by an increase in serum bicarbonate (HCO_3) concentration.

16. A: Starting the assessment with the patient's history helps establish patient rapport and build a picture of the patient's current and past respiratory problems. Inspection (B and C) and diagnostic study (D), if required, follow patient history.

17. B: Patients with emphysema typically have a barrel chest because they use their accessory muscles for breathing and sit forward to ease pressure felt in the chest. Pneumothorax (A) is accompanied by chest pain on the affected side, acute bronchitis (C) is associated with chest discomfort, and pulmonary embolism (D) can be accompanied by chest pain (pleuritic).

18. C: Blunt trauma to the ribs can be a cause of pneumothorax and should alert the nurse to this possibility. Asthma (A) can also be accompanied by chest pain, but it is not the most common symptom. Although myocardial infarction (B) is a possibility, the patient is somewhat young. Pulmonary embolism (D) typically presents with dyspnea, but it is also typically accompanied by tachypnea.

19. A: Continuous bubbling, rather than on expiration only, may point to an air leak within the system. A bubbling tube should never be clamped—this increases the risk of tension pneumothorax.

20. D: Nasal flaring occurs when breathing is labored and the patient has to do more work to breathe. Intercostal retractions are visible indentations between the ribs during breathing and are also a sign of labored breathing. Pursed lip breathing is typically seen in patients with chronic obstructive pulmonary disease and allows air to be expired slowly.

21. D: Normal respiration is typically quiet, with no use of accessory muscles, including abdomen. The normal adult respiratory range is 12 to 20 breaths/minute, and, in regular rhythm, *expiration* takes twice as long as inspiration.

22. A: Atelectasis the most common pulmonary complication of anesthesia. It involves incomplete expansion or collapse of the lung following lung compression, absorption of alveolar air, or impaired function of lung surfactant. It can follow certain types of inhaled and intravenous anesthesia. On physical examination, the nurse would expect i*ncreased* respiratory rate and *increased* pulse rate.

23. C: Maximizing ventilation and preventing aspiration are priorities until the patient can be intubated and mechanically ventilated (A). Increasing the infusion rate (B) could contribute to circulatory overload. Although oxygen therapy is a core supportive treatment, it is typically administered in high doses (>90%) via positive end-expiratory pressure (PEEP) ventilation via nasal cannula (D).

24. C: Cigarette smoking is the major risk factor for chronic bronchitis. The increased work associated with labored breathing means that patients with chronic bronchitis can be protein-deficient and lacking in muscle strength (A and B), thus diet is important, as is correct use of bronchodilators via inhaler (D).

25. C: Bronchodilators taken prior to exercise can help control or prevent EIA. Switching to an activity (A) such as swimming may reduce the likelihood of EIA being triggered. NSAIDs (B) can trigger EIA. It can be helpful to restrict exercise when feeling unwell or when allergens are high (e.g., pollen) but not avoid (D).

26. D: Although A-C play a role in decannulation according to particular hospital protocols, they are insufficient on their own to determine when or how decannulation should occur. While decannulation protocols vary, typically it involves a set of gradual changes, such as reducing tube size and cuff deflation periods, and patient monitoring.

27. D: There is no definitive study to determine pulmonary embolism (PE). D-dimer assay may indicate presence of either PE or deep venous thrombosis; chest X-ray is typically ordered but is often normal. Pulmonary angiography is the most definitive test and is typically ordered when other tests are equivocal; it shows blood flow obstruction.

28. C: The respiratory generator is composed of two groups of neurons and is located in the medulla. Chemoreceptors (A) are part of the feedback loop that adjusts respiratory center output according to blood gas levels and the diaphragm is the major muscle of inspiration. The cerebral cortex (B) exerts conscious or voluntary control over ventilation.

29. D: If obesity is a contributing factor, then weight reduction can improve sleep-disordered breathing. Continuous positive airway pressure reduces sleepiness and improves quality of life in moderate to severe obstructive sleep apnea. In some cases, medication may reduce residual

daytime sleepiness. Nocturnal monitoring is important but would typically not be conducted at home.

30. C: The pericardium is a fibrous sac that surrounds the heart and contains a small amount of fluid that reduces friction and allows the heart to change volume and size during contractions. The epicardium encases the epicardial coronary arteries (A); the chordae tendineae (B) attach the papillary to tricuspid and mitral valves; and atrioventricular valves allow unidirectional blood flow (D).

31. C: 70 to ≤90 mL/min

32. D: Tachycardia decreases left ventricular filling times.

33. A: Parasympathetic stimulation releases acetylcholine. Acetylcholine in turn decreases sinoatrial node discharge and slows conduction through atrioventricular tissue. Norepinephrine is released via sympathetic stimulation.

34. A: The bundle of His conducts impulse to the bundle branch system; the atrioventricular node delays impulse from the atria before it goes to the ventricles; the Purkinje system provides for depolarization of the myocardium.

35. D: Ventricular depolarization is represented by the QRS complex; repolarization is represented by the T wave; there is no distinctly visible wave representing atrial repolarization in the ECG because it occurs during ventricular depolarization.

36. C: CI is the CO corrected for differences in body size, based on BSA as calculated from height and weight (CI=CO/BSA). Cardiac output is the amount of blood ejected by the LV in 1 minute; ejection fraction is the percentage of blood in the ventricle ejected with every beat; BMI is a calculation of weight relative to height.

37. C: The adrenergic system is stimulatory and releases epinephrine and norepinephrine. The cholinergic system is inhibitory and releases acetylcholine. The capillary system is where tissue bed exchange of oxygen and carbon dioxide take place; the venous system receives blood from the capillaries.

38. B: Mitral stenosis can produce a low-pitched sound; neither heart failure nor atrial septal defect produce murmurs.

39. A: Radiopaque contrast medium is injected into the coronary arteries and viewed via X-ray digital imaging. EBCT is used for high-speed imaging of atherosclerosis but is limited by cost; MRI could be used in conjunction with angiography; aortography is typically used to detect aortic aneurysm.

40. D: A-C are all within the normal range for waves and intervals.

41. A: Sinus rhythm is typically 50 to 100 beats/min; sinus arrhythmia is considered if rhythm is >0.16; sinus tachycardia is considered if rate is 100 to 200 beats/min.

42. B: The ECG shows atrial activity that is chaotic, rapid, and random. Flutter waves may appear as wide, sawtooth waves; ventricular fibrillation has a bizarre, irregular waveform; and ventricular tachycardia has a wide QRS.

43. C: Dysrhythmias (A) are abnormal heart rhythms, and diaphoresis (D) is excessive sweating.

44. D: A is the Trendelenburg position; B is the Sims position; and C is the lithotomy position.

45. A: While B-D are all used to manage chronic stable angina, diuretics are not pharmacologically indicated.

46. B: Weight-adjusted heparin doses are usually changed so the APTT result is about 1.5 to 2 times the normal value (B); 30 to 40 seconds is the average normal value for partial thrombin time (PTT) (A), and 60 to 70 seconds is the average normal value for APTT (D). C is incorrect.

47. D: Left anterior descending artery.

48. A: Although fibrinolysis is effective for STEMI patients within the first 2 to 3 hours of symptom onset, it is absolutely contraindicated for patients with recent significant closed head trauma. B-D are interventions that could be used for STEMI patients.

49. B: Pacemakers have long-lasting power supplies, but it is important that the patient checks his pulse daily to make sure the pacemaker is functioning correctly. Prolonged hiccups should be reported to a physician. Pacemaker syndrome is a potential complication of an *in situ* pacemaker but not something patients can do anything to avoid.

50. C: Beta-blockers (A) reduce heart rate; stents (B) prop open arteries to improve blood flow to the heart muscle and relieve symptoms; statins (D) lower cholesterol.

51. D: Echocardiography can detect pericardial effusions, which are indicative of cardiac tamponade. Cardiac catheterization is used to detect occlusions in coronary arteries; transesophageal echocardiogram examines heart structures via a small transducer is passed down the esophagus; the Holter monitor records heartbeats on tape over a period of 24 to 48 hours during normal activities.

52. C: A is incomplete; B is metric but incorrect; D is metric but incomplete.

53. C: There is no absolute maximum dose for norepinephrine, and average doses vary across settings (though a common maximum dose is 20 mcg/min). Because norepinephrine can cause hypotension and tissue hypoxia, hemodynamic parameters need to be monitored closely.

54. B: Angioplasty increases blood flow through arteries (A) that are blocked; C is radiofrequency ablation; and cardiomyoplasty increases the pumping motion of the heart (D).

55. C: Cardiac tamponade can occur following trauma such as pacemaker insertion. This is indicated by pulsus paradoxus, a pulse that decreases in size during inhalation. Cardiac tamponade is life-threatening, and emergency pericardiocentesis is required.

56. A: Standard therapies include B-D.

57. A: B is a coarctation of the aorta; C is aortic dissection; D is aortic valve stenosis.

58. B: A is associated with peripheral arterial disease. Unlike acute MI (C), aortic dissection onset is associated with instantaneous onset of severe pain and absence of pulses. D indicates severe claudication.

59. A: Hypertension can be an underlying cause of peripheral arterial disease, and exercise therapy is the initial treatment for claudication.

60. D: Cardiogenic shock (A) is accompanied by tachycardia and pale, cool skin as a result of impaired tissue infusion. Knee surgery is a risk factor for deep venous thrombosis (DVT); in turn, DVT is the main cause of pulmonary embolism.

61. A: B is hypovolemic shock; C is neurogenic shock; and D is anaphylactic shock.

62. A: B is the normal BUN-to-creatinine ratio; C is a high BUN level, and D is a low BUN level.

63. C: A is a volume expander; B is used to treat asymptomatic hypotension and can cause pitting edema; D is a calcium channel blocker used to treat arrhythmias and can cause pitting edema.

64. A: B-C have the effect of raising blood pressure.

65. B: Complications from hypertensive crisis include cerebral, cardiac, and renal dysfunction. Low intracranial pressure typically results from head trauma or follows lumbar puncture.

66. C: Occurs during ventricular systole as a result of an incompetent mitral valve.

67. B: A and C can be caused by structural defects; D can be caused by atherosclerosis or structural defects.

68. B: Cardioversion does not cause A or C; hypokalemia is a contraindication for chemical cardioversion.

69. A: Atrial fibrillation is a supraventricular tachycardia. B-D are contraindications for pharmacologic cardioversion.

70. D: B and C are part of activating basic life protocols, which also include activating the response team.

71. C: GFR is a factor that influences sodium excretion; potassium exchange is influenced by sodium levels.

72. A: Blood urea nitrogen (BUN) measures the waste product of protein metabolism filtered and absorbed along the entire nephron, and creatinine is a waste product of muscle metabolism. Sodium concentration affects extracellular fluid (ECF) volume; potassium maintains the osmolality and electroneutrality of cells.

73. B: Oliguria is a sign of impending renal dysfunction, and initial management strategies include fluid replacement and monitoring creatinine levels, as increases indicate renal failure.

74. A: Diabetes mellitus contributes to both B and C; D is a hormonal condition in which the kidneys are unable to conserve water.

75. C: A, B, and D are all lower GI tract disorders and would be explored by other diagnostic tests such as barium enema or colonoscopy.

76. B: Hematemesis is typically sudden with varices and often projectile. A is associated with epigastric pain but not hematemesis; heartburn is a symptom of C; and D is associated with lower abdominal pain.

77. D: Sometimes referred to as "String sign." C is indicative of ulcerative colitis.

78. A: Corrects low potassium levels and high glucose levels. B is an appropriate action to correct dehydration; D is an appropriate action to correct short-term hypoglycemia.

79. D: A is basal ganglia; B is the limbic system; and C is the Circle of Willis.

80. B: A is the primary neurotransmitter of the sympathetic nervous system; C is distributed throughout the central nervous system (CNS); D is also found in the CNS.

81. C: GCS stands for Glasgow Coma Scale (score). A is part of a general assessment of neurological function; B assesses primitive reflexes associated with frontal lobe impairment; D is the assessment of a conscious, cooperative patient.

82. C: Through clipping or resection of the vessel wall. A, B, and D are used to treat arteriovenous malformations.

83. B: Complication of ischemic stroke

84. A: B-D are all complications of HIV but are not hematological.

85. B: A, C, and D are indicators of inflammation or anemia.

86. C: A, B, and D are indicators of SIRS. C should be WBC >12,000/mm³ or <4000/ mm³.

87. A: Epinephrine 0.5 mL of 1:1000 IV

88. B: A is typically the result of a surgical site infection (SSI); C is severe systemic allergic reaction with sudden onset; D is a hypersensitivity response to common allergens.

89. D: A is used to treat infection; B to treat hypotension; C to improve renal function.

90. A: Via backflow. Catheterization may be done to treat B and C; D is typically caused by blunt trauma or penetrating wound.

91. A: B can contribute to sepsis.

92. D: Establish a quiet environment, work with the patient to restore a normal sleeping pattern, and provide sleep medication.

93. B: A, C, and D could lead to unrelieved pain and delayed healing.

94. C: Tremors are a defining characteristic associated with abrupt alcohol withdrawal 12 to 48 hours following cessation; tremors are associated with delirium but not with anxiety (A), depression (B), or psychosis (D).

95. A: Benzodiazepines. Antipsychotics (B) are used to treat psychosis; Lithium (C) is used to treat manic depression; neuroleptics (D) is another term for lithium.

96. A: Restraints in progressive care are controversial though viewed as sometimes necessary. The nurse has an obligation to explore B-D before applying restraints.

97. C: Family-centered care is a philosophy that includes families as team members in the care of the patient, with the patient at the center of that approach.

98. B: A, C, and D are physician-centered rather than patient-centered.

99. C: Reflects a nurse working on behalf of the patient. A and D reflect caring practice; B reflects poor clinical judgment.

100. B: Took a long time to respond to my request.

101. D: A-C are appropriate once immediate care and safety are established.

102. B: This option addresses the boy's potential fears and reflects family-centered caring.

103. B: Combines ensuring patient warmth and comfort with human interaction and touch.

104. B: Infiltration can create complications such as pain and tissue necrosis. Identifying any reasons for repeated infiltration is an inquiry-based approach to nursing practice.

105. B: Questions the appropriateness of hospital policy and accompanies this with a patient-centered intervention and evaluation.

106. C: Questions practice based on the patient's response and suggests an alternative approach.

107. B: Helps explain the purpose of a low-fat diet.

108. A: Cardiovascular technologists assist physicians in diagnosing and treating cardiac (heart) and peripheral vascular (blood vessel) ailments; pulmonary technicians are responsible for administering pulmonary function testing.

109. A: Anemia is a complication of RA and may indicate worsening of RA.

110. A: B-D are appropriate once the patient has been informed about what the new medications are and their purpose.

111. C: This strategy incorporates individualized education into patient care, involves the family, and is based on their needs and level of understanding.

112. D: This choice uses an emergency scenario to help a newly qualified nurse learn while following emergency protocols.

113. A: This choice acknowledges differences in health beliefs while also educating the patient's family.

114. B: Telephone interpreters are available in some facilities and are trained translators that can facilitate communication in culturally diverse situations.

115. B: This choice acknowledges the importance of the patient's unique identity.

116. B: Systems thinking requires being able to see the big picture.

117. D: Discharge has been planned with the strengths and needs of the patient in mind.

118. C: Ensures that this patient's complex needs are met.

119. C: The priority nursing action for a patient arriving at the ED in distress is always assessment of vital signs. This indicates the extent of physical compromise and provides a baseline by which to plan further assessment and treatment. A thorough medical history, including onset of symptoms, will be necessary and it is likely that an electrocardiogram will be performed as well, but these are not the first priority. Similarly, chest exam with auscultation may offer useful information after vital signs are assessed.

120. C: When a family member is dying, it is most helpful for nursing staff to provide a culturally sensitive environment to the degree possible within the hospital routine. In the Vietnamese culture, it is important that the dying be surrounded by loved ones and not left alone. Traditional rituals and foods are thought to ease the transition to the next life. When possible, allowing the family privacy for this traditional behavior is best for them and the patient. A, B, and D are incorrect because they create unnecessary conflict with the patient and family.

121. D: One gel pad should be placed to the right of the sternum, just below the clavicle and the other just left of the precordium, as indicated by the anatomic location of the heart. To defibrillate, the paddles are placed over the pads. A, B, and C are not consistent with the position of the heart and are therefore incorrect responses.

122. A: A patient on nasogastric suction is at risk of metabolic alkalosis as a result of loss of hydrochloric acid in gastric fluid. Of the answers given, only answer A (pH 7.52, PCO_2 54 mm Hg) represents alkalosis. B is a normal blood gas. C represents respiratory acidosis. D is borderline normal with slightly low PCO_2.

123. A: The effect of Coumadin is to inhibit clotting. The next step is to check the PT and INR to determine the patient's anticoagulation status and risk of bleeding. Vitamin K is an antidote to Coumadin and may be used in a patient who is at imminent risk of dangerous bleeding. Preparation for transfusion, as described in option C, is only indicated in the case of significant blood loss. If lab results indicate an anticoagulation level that would place the patient at risk of excessive bleeding, the surgeon may choose to delay surgery and discontinue the medication.

124. A and B: Normal hemoglobin in adults is 12 – 16 g/dL. Total cholesterol levels of 200 mg/dL or below are considered normal. Total serum protein of 7.0-g/dL and glycosylated hemoglobin A1c of 5.4% are both normal levels.

125. A: The parathyroid glands regulate the calcium level in the blood. In hyperparathyroidism, the serum calcium level will be elevated. Parathyroid hormone levels may be high or normal but not low. The body will lower the level of vitamin D in an attempt to lower calcium. Urine calcium may be elevated, with calcium spilling over from elevated serum levels. This may cause renal stones.

Practice Test #2

Practice Questions

1. A post-MI patient is started on an angiotensin converting enzyme (ACE) inhibitor during his hospital stay. Which of the following is the most common serious side effect that may occur?
   a. Non-productive cough
   b. Pedal edema
   c. Swelling of the tongue and face
   d. Rhinorrhea

2. A patient with acute infectious diarrhea has a fever and blood in his stool. His condition does not improve with oral hydration therapy. Which of the following is a risk factor for infection with *Clostridium difficile*?
   a. Recent travel outside the U.S.
   b. History of liver transplant
   c. Daycare attendance
   d. Use of antibiotics in the past six weeks

3. In elderly patients with complaints of constipation who have no other gastrointestinal abnormalities, the initial treatment should include all of the following *except*:
   a. Stimulant laxative
   b. Increased exercise
   c. Increased fiber intake from food sources
   d. Increased water intake

4. An elderly patient with pneumonia is admitted for IV antibiotic treatment. Which of the following observations indicates that the patient may be experiencing sepsis?
   a. Productive cough
   b. Increased fluid intake
   c. Respiratory rate of 20 breaths per minute
   d. BP 90/60, HR 115 BPM

5. A nurse is evaluating a patient who had a knee replacement earlier that day. Which of the following signs is indicative of a complication of that surgery?
   a. Pain at the wound site
   b. Reluctance to bear weight on the affected leg
   c. Decreased pulses in the ankle and decreased capillary refill of the toes on the affected leg
   d. Poor appetite

6. A nurse assesses an elderly client for dementia by using the Mini-Mental Status Exam. In this exam what constitutes a score consistent with severe dementia?
   a. 24
   b. 15
   c. 28
   d. 30

7. A client is admitted with Bell's palsy. To assess the extent of the nerve involvement the nurse asks the client to:
    a. Raise eyebrows
    b. Cough
    c. Extend tongue
    d. Smile

8. Which of the following clients would most likely need surgical treatment for their fracture?
    a. 10 year old with a humeral head fracture
    b. 80 year old with a humeral midshaft fracture
    c. 40 year old with a tuft fracture of the distal phalanx
    d. 40 year old with a great toe distal phalanx fracture

9. A client with anemia is receiving an IV infusion of packed red blood cells. The client reports that they are feeling anxious and short of breath even though the respiratory rate is 20. What should the nurse do in this situation?
    a. Give a dose of lorazepam (Ativan)
    b. Give a dose of acetaminophen (Tylenol)
    c. Give a dose of diphenhydramine (Benadryl)
    d. Stop infusion and notify physician

10. An elderly client with a history of remote alcohol abuse in the past is admitted for community acquired pneumonia. In addition to usual nursing parameters what other actions are appropriate?
    a. Strict fluid intake and output
    b. Daily weights
    c. Vision checks q shift
    d. Mental status checks

11. A client comes to the ER with new onset hematemesis, a heart rate of 110 and blood pressure of 100/65. What is the first appropriate nursing intervention?
    a. Prep for NG tube
    b. Insertion of large bore peripheral IV
    c. CXR
    d. CBC

12. In outpatient diabetic management, what is the best measure of a client's glycemic control?
    a. Bun/Cr
    b. HgA1C
    c. AM blood sugar
    d. Qhs blood sugar

13. A client with chronic renal failure on dialysis misses 2 treatments due to transportation issues. The home care nurse should assess the client for which of the following:
    a. Pulmonary edema
    b. Heart murmur
    c. Temperature
    d. Gait

14. After a successful code resuscitation for asystole a client is intubated and placed on a lidocaine drip. What is the next step in care?
   a. ABG
   b. CXR for endotracheal tube placement
   c. IVF bolus
   d. Meeting of code members to discuss performance

15. A nurse assesses a client with COPD and a respiratory rate of 28. What acid-base disorder should be considered and tested for?
   a. Respiratory Acidosis
   b. Respiratory Alkalosis
   c. Metabolic Acidosis
   d. Metabolic Alkalosis

16. As part of treatment for an overdose of acetaminophen (Tylenol), a client is administered acetylcysteine (Mucomyst). What does the client need before starting this treatment?
   a. PICC line
   b. Subclavian central line
   c. Arterial line
   d. NG tube

17. Prior to performing an IV pyelogram to evaluate for kidney stones, the patient should be asked about:
   a. Prior Foley catheter use
   b. Allergies to Iodine or shellfish
   c. Recent use of antibiotics
   d. History of gallbladder disease

18. A client with renal failure has an arterio-venous shunt inserted for future dialysis. How does the nurse assess the shunt post-operatively for patency?
   a. Assess for bruit and thrill
   b. Monitor PT/PTT test results
   c. Quick flush of blood during venipuncture at site
   d. Flow during dialysis

19. A client with a history of hepatic cirrhosis is admitted for suspected spontaneous bacterial peritonitis (SBP). What area should be prepared for a culture?
   a. Lateral abdomen for ascitic fluid
   b. Lateral chest for pleural fluid
   c. Foley placement for urine
   d. Lateral abdomen for spleen biopsy

20. A client in the ER with chest pain has been judged to be a possible candidate for therapy with alteplase (tPA). Which of the following in NOT considered a contraindication for the use of this medication?
   a. Current antibiotic use
   b. Recent abdominal surgery
   c. Recent GI bleeding
   d. Recent intracranial bleed

21. Which of the following constitutes a positive PPD (Mantoux) skin test for TB?
    a. 8mm induration in a 6 year old healthy child
    b. 9 mm induration in person with HIV
    c. 4 mm induration in health care worker
    d. 3 mm induration in prison guard

22. As part of a physical exam on a client with suspected appendicitis, the physician has the client lie on the left side and extends the hip. What is the name of this maneuver?
    a. Rovsing's sign
    b. Psoas sign
    c. Kernig's sign
    d. Brudzinski's sign

23. After an outpatient surgery for knee arthroscopy, not requiring general anesthesia, a client complains of a dull headache. What is the most likely cause of the headache?
    a. Incisional pain
    b. Aneurysm
    c. Narcotic withdrawal
    d. Caffeine withdrawal

24. A client is about to have a MRI for evaluation of a possible herniated disc. What should the nurse do prior to the test?
    a. Ask about contrast dye allergy
    b. Apply large bore IV
    c. Shave lumbar area of hair
    d. Ask about prior surgery

25. In order to collect proper blood culture samples, the nurse should do which of the following?
    a. Sterilize antecubital fossa with Iodine
    b. Draw sample from femoral site
    c. Wipe culture bottles with alcohol pad
    d. Shave collection site

26. A depressed client in the mental health unit gives a visitor a 'list of things to give away'. This prompts the nurse to change his treatment plan by:
    a. Decreasing TV time
    b. Increasing group therapy time
    c. Increasing suicide precautions
    d. Increasing off-site pass time

27. A client with known hepatitis C needs to give a sputum sample. What protective gear should the nurse use in addition to gloves and a mask?
    a. Protective eyewear
    b. Shoe coverings
    c. Positive pressure respirator
    d. Earplugs

28. Following the intubation of a client with severe COPD, which usual component of mechanical ventilation is not needed?
   a. Oxygen
   b. Saturation monitoring
   c. SIMV
   d. PEEP

29. Before the initiation of chemotherapy, a 75 year old client should be assessed for all of the following areas *except*:
   a. Good bowel sounds
   b. Wounds on legs
   c. Rectal area for fissures or hemorrhoids
   d. Dentition

30. Following transfer to a Step-Down Unit from the SICU a post CABG patient should be closely monitored for:
   a. Cough
   b. Pain at sternum
   c. Increased respiratory rate
   d. Eye pain

31. Common nursing interventions for a client with acute congestive heart failure would include all of the following *except*:
   a. Remove salt from food tray
   b. Ambulate prn in halls
   c. Strict intake and output measurements of fluids
   d. Daily weights

32. Following a fall with a non-displaced rib fracture, an elderly client is instructed on the use of an incentive spirometer. The use of this aids in the prevention of:
   a. Further displacement of the fracture
   b. COPD
   c. Costochondritis
   d. Atelectasis

33. A client comes in to the clinic with a newly diagnosed infectious disease. Which of the following is NOT reportable to the health department?
   a. TB
   b. Syphilis
   c. Varicella
   d. Rabies

34. A newly diagnosed client with diabetes mellitus asks the nurse what his HbA1c level should be if he is in good control of his condition. The optimum level of HbA1c is below:
   a. 7.0
   b. 8.5
   c. 10.0
   d. 12.5

35. A client is to have a diagnostic thoracentesis. What part of the client's body should the nurse prep for the procedure?
    a. 4th rib in the mid-clavicular line
    b. 6th rib at the sternal border
    c. 7th rib in the mid-clavicular line
    d. 10th rib posteriorly

36. A client is started on allopurinol (Zyloprim) for gout. What blood test will need to be done to check for the medications efficacy?
    a. ALT
    b. HbA1c
    c. Uric acid
    d. Potassium

37. An inpatient client has a bronchial biopsy for a lung mass. What symptom indicates a possible serious complication from this procedure?
    a. Sore throat
    b. Dry cough
    c. Respiratory rate of 30
    d. Blood pressure 130/90

38. A client with hepatic encephalopathy is admitted to the hospital. What medication will likely be used to help clear this condition?
    a. Hydrochlorothiazide (HCTZ)
    b. Lactulose (Chronulac)
    c. Antacids
    d. Glycerin suppository

39. Post-operative nutritional status would be a primary concern in all of the following patients *except*:
    a. TURP
    b. Radical neck dissection
    c. Dilation of esophageal strictures
    d. Partial gastrectomy

40. Following a blood borne pathogen exposure with a needle stick a nurse decides to start post-exposure prophylaxis with antiviral medications. According to CDC guidelines how long should she take these medications?
    a. 2 days
    b. 1 year
    c. 6 months
    d. 1 month

41. A client is observed tying and untying his shoes dozens of times a day. This client is likely suffering from:
    a. Phobia
    b. PTSD
    c. OCD
    d. Depression

42. After a terminal diagnosis, a client states that he needs to be discharged because he wants to start work at a homeless shelter. What stage of grief is this client experiencing?
   a. Anger
   b. Denial
   c. Bargaining
   d. Acceptance

43. A female client is being discharged after a mastectomy for breast cancer. She expresses concern about her appearance and desirability to her husband. The nurse should:
   a. Tell her to write in a journal
   b. Speak frankly to her husband about her different appearance and their sexuality
   c. Make an appointment for a breast prosthesis
   d. Inform her that sexual activity will decrease now

44. A client in a manic state, being interviewed by a nurse, rapidly skips from one topic to the next, and does not directly answer questions. This aspect of mania is called:
   a. Heightened affect
   b. Auditory hallucinations
   c. Grandiosity
   d. Flight of ideas

45. Prior to performing an arterial blood gas (ABG) measurement on a client's hand; the nurse assesses the blood flow in the hand using what maneuver?
   a. Allen test
   b. Psoas test
   c. Rovsing's sign
   d. Kernig's sign

46. A client is discharged with a new diagnosis of severe peripheral arterial disease (PAD). In addition to medication, what should the client also have at time of discharge?
   a. Nutrition consult
   b. Smoking cessation counseling
   c. Social work consult
   d. Speech therapy consult

47. A client newly diagnosed with valvular heart disease is to be discharged from the hospital. Vital discharge instructions would include:
   a. Fertility counseling
   b. Antibiotic prophylaxis counseling
   c. Dietary modifications
   d. Social work referral

48. A nurse admits a client with possible sepsis. What is the safest and most reliable site for obtaining blood cultures?
   a. Femoral
   b. Antecubital fossa
   c. Carotid
   d. Subclavian

49. Following a fall, a client is diagnosed with a non-displaced clavicle fracture. The most likely brace to be used for this is:
   a. Thumb spica splint
   b. Elbow immobilizer
   c. Figure of 8 brace
   d. TLSO brace

50. In assessing a client with acute right-sided heart failure, which would be the most likely physical exam finding?
   a. Pedal edema
   b. Pulmonary edema
   c. Dyspnea on exertion
   d. Hepato-jugular reflex

51. An inpatient client had a colonoscopy earlier in the day. He cannot remember what the physician told him after his procedure, regarding his results. What is the most likely cause of this?
   a. GI bleeding
   b. Sedation used in procedure
   c. CVA
   d. MI

52. On a history form, a nurse notes that a client has had an enucleation of the eye in the past. What does this consist of?
   a. Removal of the eye
   b. Cataract removal
   c. Retinal repair
   d. Laser vision correction

53. An elderly client is placed on warfarin (Coumadin) for atrial fibrillation. Which of the levels listed below is a therapeutic INR level for this medication?
   a. 0.0 to 1.0
   b. 1.0 to 1.5
   c. 2.5 to 3.5
   d. 5.0 to 10.0

54. A client has a decreased respiratory rate due to an overdose of opiates. The decreased respirations put this client at risk for:
   a. Metabolic acidosis
   b. Metabolic alkalosis
   c. Respiratory acidosis
   d. Respiratory alkalosis

55. A diabetic client is counseled on the optimum blood pressure for their condition in order to minimize the risk of coronary artery disease. Normal for a diabetic is considered:
   a. 135/85
   b. 140/90
   c. 145/95
   d. 150/95

56. An elderly client is found to be dehydrated. All of the following lab values are to be expected in the initial lab results *except*:
   a. Hypernatremia
   b. Hyponatremia
   c. Increased creatinine
   d. Increased hemoglobin

57. A client is to have a bone marrow biopsy by the hematologist. What is the site that the nurse should prep for this procedure?
   a. Heel
   b. Olecranon
   c. Posterior superior pelvis
   d. Cranium

58. A client is diagnosed with new onset acute renal failure and a critically high potassium level. Until dialysis can be arranged, what medication can be used to decrease the potassium level?
   a. Sodium Polystyrene Sulfonate (Kayexalate)
   b. Furosemide (Lasix)
   c. Benazepril (Lotensin)
   d. Hydrochlorothiazide (HCTZ)

59. An elderly client is diagnosed with *Clostridium difficile* colitis. What is the most likely cause of this condition?
   a. Travel to a tropical state
   b. MI
   c. IV antibiotic use for pneumonia
   d. Drinking unfiltered water from a stream

60. A client with community-acquired pneumonia needs antibiotic treatment. The client has a severe penicillin allergy. What would be the best treatment for this client?
   a. Benzathine penicillin (Bicillin LA)
   b. Nafcillin (Nallpen)
   c. Azithromycin (Zithromax)
   d. Amoxicillin (Amoxil)

61. Following a fall on the elbow joint a client is noted to have a swollen elbow and the inability to fully extend the joint. The most likely fracture is:
   a. Radial head fracture
   b. Colles' fracture
   c. Smith's fracture
   d. Scaphoid fracture

62. An elderly client on warfarin therapy has an INR level of 5.5. What vitamin can be used to counteract the effects of the medication and decrease the risk of bleeding?
    a. Vitamin A
    b. Vitamin B12
    c. Vitamin C
    d. Vitamin K

63. Which of the following GI conditions may also involve the esophagus?
    a. Crohn's disease
    b. Diverticulitis
    c. Diverticulosis
    d. Ulcerative colitis

64. All of the following can cause atrial fibrillation at high doses *except*:
    a. Alcohol
    b. Caffeine
    c. Acetaminophen (Tylenol)
    d. Cocaine

65. An elderly client with an abdominal aortic aneurysm (AAA) declines surgery for the condition. What medication may be beneficial in prevention of rupture of this aneurysm?
    a. Benazepril (Lotensin)
    b. Captopril (Capoten)
    c. Metoprolol (Toprol)
    d. Ramipril (Altace)

66. At the time of admission, clients with pancreatitis are often classified to determine mortality risk using the Ranson criteria. Which of the following is NOT part of the Ranson criteria staging?
    a. Age
    b. WBC
    c. Sex
    d. Blood sugar

67. Following a CVA a client is noted to understand speech but have difficulty with expressing words to communicate. This is known as:
    a. Expressive aphasia
    b. Echolalia
    c. Pressured speech
    d. Cerebral palsy

68. The Thompson test is used to assess the functionality of what body part?
    a. Quadriceps
    b. Elbow
    c. Shoulder
    d. Achilles tendon

69. Rank the following interventions for use during a code resuscitation for ventricular fibrillation in terms of time used (most important used first):
   a. Lidocaine
   b. Defibrillation
   c. Epinephrine
   d. Sodium bicarbonate

70. During treatment of ventricular tachycardia, what medication is given via IV push that frequently results in a brief asystolic episode?
   a. Lidocaine
   b. Epinephrine
   c. Adenosine
   d. Bretylium

71. Which of the following areas on a 70 year old client affected by a herpes zoster (shingles) rash, is likely to need IV antiviral therapy to avoid serious complications?
   a. Dorsal hand
   b. Groin
   c. Neck
   d. Temple

72. A client is scheduled to have a treadmill stress ECG test for a cardiac evaluation. Which of the following is NOT considered a contraindication for the testing?
   a. History of MI one year ago
   b. BP 190/122
   c. Aortic stenosis
   d. Pulmonary edema

73. A client in the hospital receiving IV antibiotics for pneumonia states that he wishes to leave the hospital and does not want any further treatment. His physician is unavailable to speak to the client. What is the next proper step for the nurse?
   a. Notify the local police
   b. Have security restrain the client in the room
   c. Have the client sign an against medical advice (AMA) form and allow him to leave
   d. Engage other nursing staff to try and convince the client to stay

74. A client is found to have a complete transection of the spinal cord at L3. Which of the following actions would the client most likely be unable to perform?
   a. Flex knee
   b. Flex hips
   c. Adduct shoulders
   d. Extend wrists

75. A client is to be given 750 mg of a medication IV. The medication comes in a vial with 200 mg/ml. How many ml does the client need?
   a. 3.05 ml
   b. 3.75 ml
   c. 3.85 ml
   d. 3.95 ml

76. A client weighs 125 kg. The client is to start an IV medication that is dosed at 60 mg/kg/day divided tid. What dose should the client be given?
    a. 1550 mg IV tid
    b. 2500 mg IV tid
    c. 1500 mg IV tid
    d. 2550 mg IV tid

77. A central venous pressure reading of 11cm/H(2)0 of an IV of normal saline is determined by the nurse caring for the patient. The patient has a diagnosis of pericarditis. Which of the following is the most applicable:
    a. The patient has a condition of hypovolemia
    b. Not enough fluid has been given to the patient
    c. Pericarditis may cause pressures greater than 10cm/H(2)0 with testing of CVP
    d. The patient may have a condition of arteriosclerosis

78. A nurse reviewed the arterial blood gas reading of a 25 year-old male. The nurse should be able to conclude the patient is experiencing which of the following conditions?
Bicarbonate ion-25 mEq/l
PH-7.41
PaCO2-29 mmHg
PaO2-54 mmHg
(FiO2)-.22
    a. metabolic acidosis
    b. respiratory acidosis
    c. metabolic alkalosis
    d. respiratory alkalosis

79. Medical records indicate a patient has developed a condition of respiratory alkalosis. Which of the following clinical signs would not apply to a condition of respiratory alkalosis?
    a. Muscle tetany
    b. Syncope
    c. Numbness
    d. Anxiety

80. Which of the following lab values would indicate symptomatic AIDS in the medical chart? (T4 cell count per deciliter)
    a. Greater than 1000 cells per deciliter
    b. Less than 500 cells per deciliter
    c. Greater than 2000 cells per deciliter
    d. Less than 200 cells per deciliter

81. A nurse notices a mole with irregular edges with a bluish color. The nurse should:
    a. Recommend a dermatological consult to the MD
    b. Note the location of the mole and contact the physician via the telephone
    c. Note the location of the mole and follow-up with the attending physician via the medical record and phone call
    d. Remove the mole with a sharp's debridement technique, following charge nurse approval

82. A nurse taking a patient's history realizes the patient is complaining of SOB and weakness in the lower extremities. The patient has a history of hyperlipidemia, and hypertension. Which of the following may be occurring?
   a. The patient is developing CHF
   b. The patient may be having a MI
   c. The patient may be developing COPD
   d. The patient may be having an onset of PVD

83. A nurse has been assigned a patient who has recently been diagnosed with Guillain-Barre' Syndrome. Which of the following statements is the most applicable when discussing the impairments with Guillain-Barre' Syndrome with the patient?
   a. Guillain-Barre' Syndrome gets better after 5 years in almost all cases
   b. Guillain-Barre' Syndrome causes limited sensation in the abdominal region
   c. Guillain-Barre' Syndrome causes muscle weakness in the legs
   d. Guillain-Barre' Syndrome does not affect breathing in severe cases

84. A doctor tells you a patient is exhibiting signs of right-sided heart failure. Which of the following would not indicate right-sided heart failure?
   a. Nausea
   b. Anorexia
   c. Rapid weight gain
   d. SOB (shortness of breath)

85. A nurse is reviewing a patient's ECG report. The patient exhibits a flat T wave, depressed ST segment and short QT interval. Which of the following medications can cause all of the above effects?
   a. Morphine
   b. Atropine
   c. Procardia
   d. Digitalis

86. A patient has recently been diagnosed with symptomatic bradycardia. Which of the following medications is the most recognized for treatment of symptomatic bradycardia?
   a. Questran
   b. Digitalis
   c. Nitroglycerin
   d. Atropine

87. A patient has recently been prescribed Lidocaine Hydrochloride. Which of the following symptoms may occur with over dosage?
   a. Memory loss and lack of appetite
   b. Confusion and fatigue
   c. Heightened reflexes
   d. Tinnitus and spasticity

88. A patient has recently been prescribed Albuterol. Which of the following changes are not associated with Albuterol?
    a. Tachycardia
    b. Hypertension
    c. Bronchodilation
    d. Sensory changes

89. Which of the following arterial blood gas values indicates a patient may be experiencing a condition of metabolic acidosis?
    a. PaO2 (90%)
    b. Bicarbonate 15.9 mmol/L
    c. CO(2) 47 mm Hg
    d. pH 7.34

90. A patient has a history of cardiac arrhythmia. A nurse has been ordered to give 2 units of blood to this patient. The nurse should take which of the following actions?
    a. Prep the patient with pain medication
    b. Notify the patient's family about the procedure via the telephone
    c. Decrease the temperature of the blood to be given
    d. Increase the temperature of the blood to be given

91. A nurse is reviewing a patient's serum glucose levels. Which of the following scenarios would indicate abnormal serum glucose values for a 30 year-old male?
    a. 70 mg/dl
    b. 55 mg/dl
    c. 110 mg/dl
    d. 100 mg/dl

92. A nurse is reviewing a patient's current Lithium levels. Which of the following values is outside the therapeutic range?
    a. 1.0 mEq/L
    b. 1.1 mEq/L
    c. 1.2 mEq/L
    d. 1.3 mEq/L

93. A nurse has been ordered to set-up Buck's traction on a patient's lower extremity due to a femur fracture. Which of the following applies to Buck's traction?
    a. A weight greater than 10 lbs. should be used
    b. The line of pull is upward at an angle
    c. The line of pull is straight
    d. A weight greater than 20 lbs. should be used

94. A nurse is caring for a patient who has experienced burns to the right lower extremity. According to the Rule of Nines which of the following percents most accurately describes the severity of the injury?
    a. 36%
    b. 27%
    c. 18%
    d. 9%

95. Which of the following is not considered one of the five rights of medication administration?
    a. client
    b. drug
    c. dose
    d. routine

96. A nurse gave medications to the wrong client. She stated the client responded to the name called. What is the nurse's appropriate documentation?
    a. Note in medication records the drug given
    b. The client was not hurt, no need for documentation
    c. Note the client's orientation
    d. Completely fill out an incident report

97. If your patient is acutely psychotic, which of the following independent nursing interventions would not be appropriate?
    a. Conveying calmness with one on one interaction
    b. Recognizing and dealing with your own feelings to prevent escalation of the
    c. patient's anxiety level
    d. Encourage client participation in group therapy
    e. Listen and identify causes of their behavior

98. You are responsible for reviewing the med. refrigerator. If you found the following drug in the refrigerator it should be removed from the refrigerator's contents?
    a. Corgard
    b. Humulin (injection)
    c. Urokinase
    d. Epogen (injection)

99. A nurse has just suffered a needlestick while working with a patient that is positive for AIDS. Which of the following is the most important action that nurse should take?
    a. Immediately see a social worker
    b. Start prophylactic AZT treatment
    c. Start prophylactic Pentamide treatment
    d. Seek counseling

100. A thirty five year old male has been an insulin-dependent diabetic for five years and now is unable to urinate. Which of the following would you most likely suspect?
    a. Atherosclerosis
    b. Diabetic nephropathy
    c. Autonomic neuropathy
    d. Somatic neuropathy

101. A nurse is caring for an adult that has recently been diagnosed with renal failure. Which of the following clinical signs would most likely not be present?
    a. Hypotension
    b. Heart failure
    c. Dizziness
    d. Memory loss

102. The nurse is caring for a client following an appendectomy. The client reports nausea and complains of surgical site pain at a 6 on a 0 to 10 scale. The client's employer is present in the room and states he is paying for the insurance and wants to know what pain medication has been prescribed by the physician. Which of the following is the appropriate nurse response?
   a. Answer any questions the employer may have as he pays for the insurance
   b. Tell the employer his question is inappropriate and that the information is none of his business
   c. Explain to the employer that you cannot release private information and ask the employer to step out while you conduct your assessment of the client
   d. Ask the employer to leave and wait until the client returns home to visit

103. When assessing a client with glaucoma, a nurse expects which of the following findings?
   a. Complaints of double vision
   b. Complaints of halos around lights
   c. Intraocular pressure of 15 mm Hg
   d. Soft globe on palpation

104. While undergoing hemodialysis, the client becomes restless and tells the nurse he has a headache and feels nauseous. Which of the following complications does the nurse suspect?
   a. Infection
   b. Disequilibrium syndrome
   c. Air embolus
   d. Acute hemolysis

105. The nurse is caring for a 44-year-old client diagnosed with hypoparathyroidism. Which electrolyte imbalance is closely associated with hypoparathyroidism?
   a. Hypocalcemia
   b. Hyponatremia
   c. Hyperkalemia
   d. Hypophosphatemia

106. The nurse is checking laboratory values on a patient who has crackling rales in the lower lobes, 2+ pitting edema, and dyspnea with minimal exertion. Which of the following laboratory values does the nurse expect to be abnormal?
   a. Potassium
   b. B-type natriuretic peptide (BNP)
   c. C-reactive protein (CRP)
   d. Platelets

107. A nurse is taking the health history of an 85-year-old client. Which of the following physical findings is consistent with normal aging?
   a. Increase in subcutaneous fat
   b. Diminished cough reflex
   c. Long-term memory loss
   d. Myopia

108. The nurse is caring for a client after a lung lobectomy. The nurse notes fluctuating water levels in the water-seal chamber of the client's chest tube. What action should the nurse take?
   a. Do nothing, but continue to monitor the client
   b. Call the physician immediately
   c. Check the chest tube for a loose connection
   d. Add more water to the water-seal chamber

109. The nurse is preparing to administer an I.M. injection in a client with a spinal cord injury that has resulted in paraplegia. Which of the following muscles is best site for the injection in this case?
   a. Deltoid
   b. Dorsal gluteal
   c. Vastus lateralis
   d. Ventral gluteal

110. The nurse is caring for a client with heart failure. Which of the following statements by the client suggests that the client has left-sided heart failure?
   a. "I sleep on three pillows each night."
   b. "My feet are bigger than normal."
   c. "My pants don't fit around my waist."
   d. "I have to get up three times during the night to urinate."

111. The nurse is assessing a client with aortic stenosis. Which of the following best describes the murmur associated with aortic stenosis?
   a. High-pitched and blowing
   b. Loud and rough during systole
   c. Low-pitched, rumbling during diastole
   d. Low-pitched and blowing

112. The nurse is caring for a client with pulmonary edema. Which of the following orders should the nurse clarify?
   a. Dobutamine 5 mcg/kg/minute I.V.
   b. 0.9% normal saline solution I.V. at 150 mL/hour
   c. Morphine I.V. 2 mg every 2 hours P.R.N. dyspnea
   d. Furosemide I.V. 40 mg every 6 hours

113. The nurse is caring for a client with cirrhosis of the liver. The client has developed ascites and requires a paracentesis. Which of the following symptoms is associated with ascites and should be relieved by the paracentesis?
   a. Pruritus
   b. Dyspnea
   c. Jaundice
   d. Peripheral neuropathy

114. A client is admitted to the medical-surgical floor with a diagnosis of acute pancreatitis. His blood pressure is 136/76 mm Hg, pulse 96 beats/minute, respirations 22 breaths/minute, temperature 99°F (38.3°C), and he has been experiencing severe vomiting for 24 hours. His past medical history reveals hyperlipidemia and alcohol abuse. The physician prescribes a nasogastric (NG) tube for the client. Which of the following is the primary purpose for insertion of the NG tube?
   a. Empty the stomach of fluids and gas to relieve vomiting
   b. Prevent spasms at the sphincter of Oddi
   c. Prevent air from forming in the small and large intestines
   d. Remove bile from the gallbladder

115. The nurse is caring for a client who requires a nasogastric (NG) tube for feeding. What should the nurse do immediately after inserting an NG tube for enteral feedings?
   a. Aspirate for gastric secretions with a syringe
   b. Begin feeding slowly to prevent cramping
   c. Get an X-ray of the tip of the tube within 24 hours
   d. Clamp off the tube until the feedings begin

116. A client is experiencing an acute episode of ulcerative colitis. Which of the following is the most important nursing action for this client?
   a. Replace lost fluid and sodium
   b. Monitor for increased serum glucose level from steroid therapy
   c. Restrict the dietary intake of foods high in potassium
   d. Note any change in the color and consistency of stools

117. A client who recently underwent cranial surgery develops syndrome of inappropriate antidiuretic hormone (SIADH). Which of the following symptoms should the nurse anticipate?
   a. Edema and weight gain
   b. Excessive urinary output
   c. Fluid loss and dehydration
   d. Low urine specific gravity

118. The nurse is assessing a client with chronic bronchospasm, which is treated with oral theophylline. Which of the following serum theophylline levels requires immediate nursing action?
   a. 8 μg/mL
   b. 12 μg/mL
   c. 20 μg/mL
   d. 25 μg/mL

119. A client is admitted with acute pancreatitis. Which of the following laboratory results is expected for this client?
   a. Serum creatinine of 4.3 mg/dL
   b. Alanine aminotransferase (ALT) of 125 IU/L
   c. Serum amylase of 306 IU/L
   d. Troponin T level of 3.5 μg/L

120. A client suddenly becomes short of breath. Which position is most beneficial for a client experiencing respiratory difficulty?
   a. Dorsal recumbent
   b. Lithotomy
   c. Semi-Fowler's
   d. Sims'

121. A client is admitted with a possible bowel obstruction. Which of the following nursing actions is most important for the nurse to perform for a client with a bowel obstruction?
   a. Obtain daily weights
   b. Measure abdominal girth
   c. Keep strict intake and output
   d. Encourage the client to increase fluids

122. The nurse is caring for a client diagnosed with a stroke. Because of the stroke, the client has dysphagia (difficulty swallowing). Which intervention by the nurse is best for preventing aspiration?
   a. Placing the client in high Fowler's position to eat
   b. Offering liquids and solids together
   c. Keeping liquids thinned
   d. Placing food on the affected side of the mouth

123. The nurse is caring for a client who suddenly develops a tonic-clonic seizure. Which nursing action is most appropriate during a seizure?
   a. Forcing a padded tongue blade into the client's mouth
   b. Restraining the client's limbs
   c. Placing the client in a supine position
   d. Loosening constrictive clothing

124. A client has just returned from the X-ray department, where a cervical myelogram with a water-based dye was performed. Which of the following interventions does the nurse include after this procedure?
   a. Force fluids
   b. Monitor blood glucose level for 24 hours
   c. Maintain the client flat in bed for 12 hours
   d. Turn the client from side to side after 2 hours

125. A client was admitted 3 days earlier with a suspected brain tumor. During assessment, the nurse notes clear drainage from the nose. Which action by the nurse may help to determine whether the drainage is cerebrospinal fluid (CSF)?
   a. Test the pH of the drainage
   b. Test the drainage for glucose
   c. Observe the drainage for a brown stain
   d. Test the specific gravity of the drainage

Answers and Explanations

1. C: Although A, B, and D are side effects seen with newly started ACE inhibitors, edema of the tongue and face can be severe enough to require intubation and respirator use. Patients should be instructed to not ignore any signs of swelling in the tongue and face and seek medical attention immediately.

2. D: The use of antibiotics in the past six weeks is a risk factor for *Clostridium difficile*. Antibiotic use disrupts the normal flora of the bowel leading to overgrowth by *C. difficile* with the release of toxins and resulting in inflammation.

3. A: Answers B, C, and D are all first line treatments for constipation in the elderly. Stimulant laxatives should be avoided as they can lead to dependence and irregularity in the gastrointestinal tract.

4. D: Dropping blood pressure and rising heart rate indicate that the patient may be getting septic. Notification of the physician and ICU transfer is advisable.

5. C: Decreased pulses and capillary refill indicate a possible injury to the posterior tibial artery during surgery. Immediate evaluation by the surgeon is warranted.

6. B: The MMSE is a test given to assess mental status and has a best score of 30/30. Any score less than 16 would indicate severe dementia.

7. D: Bell's palsy affects the seventh cranial nerve. By asking the patient to smile, the nurse could observe evidence of the condition. The client would have a droop in the facial expression on the side involved.

8. A: A 10 year old would need operative treatment for a humeral head fracture that would possibly impair future growth and development. The treatments for the situations in Answers C and D would be splinting and Answer B would require a sling.

9. D: Anxiety and the sensation of breathlessness are signs of possible anaphylactic shock, the infusion should be stopped immediately, and the physician notified.

10. D: Withdrawal from alcohol can lead to delirium tremens and can be possibly fatal. Even if a client denies current use of alcohol it is prudent to monitor mental status for any signs of deterioration. Benzodiazepines can be used for blunt withdrawals.

11. B: In a patient with potential shock due to blood loss, the most important intervention is fluid resuscitation. Large bore IVs should be inserted first.

12. B: The best measure of long term glycemic control is HgA1c. This gives an evaluation of a client's glycemic control for the past 3 months and is the best guide for future medication choices.

13. A: In addition to clearance of toxins, dialysis also clears excess fluid. The client should be assessed for fluid overload, because if pulmonary edema is present it may require urgent dialysis.

14. B: After any intubation, a CXR is vital to insure proper placement. Even with good breath sounds on both sides and CO_2 monitoring, a CXR is essential.

15. B: A rapid respiratory rate will lead to a loss of CO_2 and a respiratory alkalosis. No metabolic process is involved.

16. D: Mucomyst is given via NG tube and this must be in place before starting treatment.

17. B: Patients with an allergy to Iodine or shellfish often also have an allergy to contrast dye that would be used in this test. Should this be present, premedication or an alternate test may be necessary.

18. A: Assessing for a bruit and thrill are the methods of evaluating patency of an AV shunt. Venipunctures and blood pressure cuffs should never be used on that arm.

19. A: Infection of ascites fluid is the cause of SBP and a specimen will need to be taken from this for culture.

20. A: Use of antibiotics is not a contraindication for use of t-PA. Recent abdominal surgery, GI bleeding and intracranial bleed are all contraindications for use of this medication.

21. B: Any induration over 5 mm in a person with immunosuppression is considered a positive test. A health care worker or prison guard would be considered to have a positive test with over 10mm induration and a healthy client with no risk factors would have a positive test with over 15mm induration.

22. B: Pain with extension of the hip is known as the psoas sign and it indicates irritation to the posterior peritoneal space by the inflamed appendix. Answers C and D deal with meningitis and answer A is pain in the RLQ elicited after pressing on the LLQ.

23. D: The most commonly used drug in the United States is caffeine. As clients are kept NPO for outpatient procedures withdrawal from morning caffeine is a very common cause of headaches in the ambulatory arena.

24. D: The client should be asked about prior surgical procedures that may have left metallic screws or plates. A MRI can move these and may not be safe. No dye in used in an MRI and no IV or shaving is needed.

25. A: In order to minimize contaminants, blood cultures are taken from the antecubital fossa after sterilizing with iodine and using sterile gloves.

26. C: The giving away of possessions is a sign of an impending suicide attempt, the patients activities should be monitored more closely and the physician in charge notified.

27. A: Coughing can aerosolize saliva, which may contain the hepatitis C virus. Protective eyewear would be recommended.

28. D: A client with COPD will have retention of air in the lungs and PEEP (positive end expiratory pressure) is not needed. Oxygen, saturation monitoring, and SIMV are all needed.

29. A: Before initiation of chemotherapy that may potentially immunosuppress a client, possible sites of infection should be addressed.

30. C: Following a major cardiac surgery and extubation, an increase in respiratory rate may signal worsening of condition and impending respiratory collapse.

31. B: Unless allowed by physician physical activity should be limited until the patient improves. Options A, C, and D are all standard interventions for such a patient.

32. D: An incentive spirometer encourages deep breathing and decreases the risk of atelectasis, which can lead to fever and pneumonia.

33. C: The other three answers are all reportable diseases to the local health department. The varicella virus, which causes chicken pox, is not.

34. A: For a client to be in good control of their diabetes their HgA1c level needs to be under 7.0. Any level higher than that may indicate a necessity in changing or increasing medication.

35. D: For a diagnostic thoracentesis, a needle is inserted over a rib to draw fluid and, to prevent damage to underlying structures, it is usually done in the posterior thorax area.

36. C: Gout is caused by the pathologic increase in uric acid level due to an enzyme deficiency. Allopurinol is used to decrease the uric acid level and prevent future attacks.

37. C: The most common serious complication of a bronchial biopsy is a pneumothorax which would be initially evident with dyspnea and an increased respiratory rate.

38. B: Lactulose is used to cleanse the colon of ammonia increasing bacteria. Through the reduction in the ammonia levels in the blood, the symptoms of encephalopathy resolve.

39. A: Smoking increases the risk of DVT and heart disease in women taking oral contraceptive pills. Smokers should be offered other choices first.

40. D: According to CDC guidelines, it is advisable for the exposed employee to take anti-viral medication for one month to decrease the potential risk of HIV conversion.

41. C: The repetitive performance of an act is a key component of obsessive-compulsive disorder (OCD). The client repeats the act until they feel it is "just right" or until it relieves their anxiety.

42. C: This client is in that bargaining stage of grief and likely feels that if he performs enough good deeds that it may alter his diagnosis.

43. B: With any change in body image, it is imperative for the client to speak with her husband and maintain an open dialogue.

44. D: The rapid skipping between topics is a classic aspect of mania. Although the other answers may be a part of a manic state, the question deals with this aspect of speech.

45. A: The Allen test is used to test collateral circulation in the hand before performing an ABG sampling. The psoas and Rovsing's signs are tests for appendicitis and Kernig's sign is a test for meningitis.

46. B: Cessation of tobacco use is the most important non-pharmacologic intervention that can be done to improve PAD.

47. B: A client with valvular heart disease must be counseled to arrange for antibiotic prophylaxis before any invasive medical procedure in the future in order to prevent bacterial endocarditis. This includes dental procedures and many diagnostic tests.

48. B: The safest area and one least likely to have contaminants is the antecubital fossa. Venipuncture in the carotid and subclavian area are potentially dangerous and due to risk of contamination, the femoral site is not advised.

49. C: A figure 8 brace is used to keep the shoulders in good positioning for healing of the clavicle. The other braces are not used for clavicle fractures.

50. D: Right-sided heart failure leads to congestion in the venous return areas of the body. Pedal and pulmonary edema and dyspnea on exertion are all findings consistent with left sided heart failure.

51. B: Benzodiazepines are commonly used as sedation during colonoscopies. Short-term memory loss is a common side-effect and the patient needs another visit by the physician to go over his results.

52. A: Enucleation involves the complete removal of the eye. It is usually performed after severe trauma or cancer.

53. C: The therapeutic INR bleeding time for a client on anticoagulation therapy with warfarin is 2.5 to 3.5. This needs to be monitored periodically during treatment.

54. C: Due to the inability to breathe off carbon dioxide a respiratory acidosis may ensue. There is no metabolic process at work.

55. A: Although 140/90 may be considered normal for most in the population, 135/85 is considered the upper limit of normal for diabetics

56. B: With dehydration, electrolyte levels and blood counts may be elevated due to decreased circulating blood volume. Thus, hypernatremia, and increased creatinine and hemoglobin would be found but not hyponatremia.

57. C: The posterior aspect of the pelvis is the site most commonly used for assessment in bone marrow biopsies.

58. A: Kayexalate is a medication used to bind potassium and clear it from the body. It can be used short term in order to decrease potassium levels from dangerous levels while awaiting dialysis treatment.

59. C: *C. difficile* most commonly arises when antibiotic use causes a disruption of the normal bowel flora giving the pathogenic organisms the ability to rapidly multiply and cause colitis.

60. C: Zithromax is a macrolide antibiotic and would not likely cause an allergy in penicillin- allergic individuals. The other answers are all derivatives in the penicillin family and should be avoided.

61. A: These symptoms are classic for radial head fracture. This fracture may not be evident initially on x-ray and may need to be reimaged in one week. The other answers are all wrist fractures.

62. D: The mechanism of action of warfarin is as an antagonist of vitamin K and this vitamin can be used to correct an overmedicated client.

63. A: Crohn's disease can involve any part of the digestive system from mouth to anus. The other answers are all limited to the colon.

64. C: In high doses, Tylenol does not greatly increase the risk of atrial fibrillation. The other answers all are known to increase the risk of arrhythmias at high doses.

65. C: Beta-blockers such as metoprolol may be beneficial in the prevention of rupture of an AAA. The other answers are ACE inhibitors and would not have this benefit.

66. C: Age, WBC, blood sugar, LDH and ALT levels are all used to stratify mortality risk. Sex is not a factor.

67. A: Impairment in vocalizing is known as an expressive aphasia and is often seen with CVAs that involve the left side of the cerebrum.

68. D: The Thompson test consists of squeezing a client's calf while they are in the prone position to assess for Achilles tendon rupture. An intact tendon will result in extension of the foot.

69. Answer: B, C, A, D is the proper order. In ventricular fibrillation, the most important intervention is defibrillation followed by epinephrine and then lidocaine. Sodium bicarbonate is used occasionally after long codes.

70. C: Adenosine is used in the treatment of some ventricular tachycardias and is given via IV push. A brief asystolic episode is common.

71. D: A herpes zoster rash on the temple area may develop into involvement of the eye and can lead to blindness. It should be treated with IV antivirals to prevent this complication.

72. A: MI is not a contraindication for treadmill stress ECG testing, and stress tests are often used as diagnostic procedures in these patients. The other answers are all contraindications to stress testing.

73. C: Unless the client is admitted via a court order, if competent, they can leave at any time. It is advisable to have them sign the AMA form to reduce liability risk on the institution.

74. A: Flexion of the knee is performed with the hamstrings which are innervated by L4, L5, S1, and Sb. Transection at L3 would eliminate this ability.

75. Answer: 3.75 ml. By multiplying 750 mg by 1ml/200 mg we get an answer of 3.75 ml.

76. Answer: 2500 mg IV tid. By using 125 kg x 60 mg/kg, we get a total dose of 7500 mg/day. As this is to be given tid, we divide 7500 mg by 3 and get 2500 mg IV.

77. C: >10cm/H(2)0 may indicate a condition of pericarditis

78. D: Respiratory alkalosis-elevated pH, and low carbon dioxide levels, no compensation noted

79. D: Anxiety is a clinical sign associated with respiratory acidosis.

80. D: <200 T4 cells/deciliter

81. C: Contacting the attending physician via the medical record is appropriate due to the possibility of melanoma.

82. B: Myocardial infarction may be associated with SOB and muscle weakness.

83. C: Muscle weakness in the lower extremities is found in acute cases of Guillain-Barre' Syndrome.

84. D: Left-sided heart failure exhibits signs of pulmonary compromise (SOB).

85. D: Digitalis can cause all of the listed symptoms.

86. D: Atropine encourages increased rate of conduction in the AV node.

87. B: Lidocaine Hydrochloride can cause fatigue and confusion if an over dosage occurs.

88. D: Tachycardia, hypertension, and bronchodilation can all occur with Albuterol.

89. B: The bicarbonate value is below normal, indicating a condition of metabolic acidosis.

90. D: Warming the blood will reduce the risk of additional cardiac arrhythmia.

91. B: 60-115 mg/dl is standard range for serum glucose levels.

92. D: 1.0-1.2 mEq/L is considered standard therapeutic range for patient care.

93. C: A straight line of pull is indicated with Buck's traction.

94. C: Each lower extremity is scored as 18% according to the Rule of Nines.

95. D: Dose, client, drug, route and time are considered the five rights of medication.

96. D: The incident report should always be filled out involving medication errors.

97. C: Acutely psychotic patients will disrupt group activities.

98. A: Corgard could be removed from the refrigerator.

99. B: AZT treatment is the most critical intervention.

100. C: Autonomic neuropathy can cause inability to urinate.

101. A: Hypertension is often related renal failure.

102. C: Explaining to the employer that the nurse cannot release information and asking the employer to step out while conducting an assessment allows the client privacy while still being respectful of the employer. Although the employer is paying for the insurance, this does not given him a right to confidential information. Providing information to the client's employer without permission is a violation of the right to privacy under HIPAA. Speaking rudely to a visitor by saying something is "none of his business" is never appropriate. Asking the person to leave and to wait until the client returns home to visit wrongly assumes the nurse has the right to speak for the patient.

103. B: A complaint of halos around lights is a common finding in a client with glaucoma. Symptoms of glaucoma don't include double vision but can include loss of peripheral vision or blind spots, reddened sclera, firm globe, decreased accommodation, and occasional eye pain, but clients may be asymptomatic until permanent damage to the optic nerve and retina has occurred. Normal intraocular pressure is 10 to 21 mm Hg.

104. B: Disequilibrium syndrome is caused by a rapid reduction in urea, sodium, and other solutes from the blood. This may lead to cerebral edema and increased intracranial pressure (ICP). Signs and symptoms of increased ICP include headache, nausea, and restlessness as well as vomiting, confusion, twitching, and seizures. Fever and an elevated white blood cell count may indicate infection. Popping or ringing in the ears, chest pain, dizziness, or coughing suggests an air embolus. Chest pain, dyspnea, burning at the access site, and cramping suggest acute hemolysis.

105. A: The parathyroid glands are responsible for maintaining calcium levels at 8.8 to 10.2 mg/dL. In hypoparathyroidism, parathyroid hormone levels are insufficient to maintain adequate calcium levels. The nurse should monitor clients with hypoparathyroidism for signs and symptoms of hypocalcemia, including muscle spasms, anxiety, seizures, hypotension, and congestive heart failure. Hyponatremia and hyperkalemia aren't associated with hypoparathyroidism. Hyperphosphatemia, not hypophosphatemia, may be seen in the client with hypoparathyroidism as calcium levels decrease.

106. B: The client's symptoms suggest heart failure. BNP is a neurohormone that is released from the ventricles when the ventricles experience increased pressure and stretch, such as in heart failure. A BNP level greater than 51 pg/mL is often associated with mild heart failure; and, as the BNP level increases, the severity of heart failure increases. Potassium levels are not affected by heart failure. CRP is an indicator of inflammation. It is used to help predict the risk of coronary artery disease. There is no indication that the client has an increased CRP. There is no indication that the client is experiencing bleeding or clotting abnormalities, such as those seen with an abnormal platelet count.

107. B: Diminished cough reflex is consistent with normal aging, putting older adults at increased risk for aspiration and atelectasis. A decrease in subcutaneous fat increases risk for pressure ulcers. Long-term memory is usually intact unless the client suffers from dementia, but short-term

memory is often impaired. Presbyopia (far-sightedness) is common with aging. Those who have had myopia (near-sightedness) may find their vision improving with age.

108. A: Fluctuation in the water-seal chamber is a normal finding that occurs as the client breathes. No action is required except for continued monitoring of the client. The nurse doesn't need to notify the physician. Continuous bubbling in the water-seal chamber indicates an air leak in the chest tube system, such as from a loose connection in the chest tube tubing. The water-seal chamber should be filled initially to the 2 cm line, and no more water should be added.

109. A: I.M. injections should be given in the deltoid muscle in the client with a spinal cord injury. Paraplegia involves paralysis and lack of sensation in the lower trunk and lower extremities. Clients with spinal cord injuries exhibit reduced use of and consequently reduced blood flow to muscles in the buttocks (dorsal gluteal and ventral gluteal) and legs (vastus lateralis). Decreased blood flow results in impaired drug absorption and increases the risk of local irritation and trauma, which could result in ulceration of the tissue.

110. A: Orthopnea is a classic sign of left-sided heart failure. The client often sleeps on several pillows at night to help facilitate breathing because of pulmonary edema. Peripheral edema is indicative or right-sided failure. Ascites is a late symptom of right-sided heart failure and can increase girth. Nocturia is common with right-sided failure as peripheral edema decreases when the feet are not dependent, increasing urinary output.

111. B: An aortic murmur is loud and rough and is heard over the aortic area during systole. Aortic insufficiency has a high-pitched and blowing murmur and is heard at the third or fourth intercostal space at the left sternal border. Mitral stenosis has a low-pitched rumbling murmur heard at the apex. Mitral insufficiency has a high-pitched, blowing murmur at the apex. There is no specific condition associated with a low-pitched, blowing murmur.

112. B: An I.V. rate of 150 mL/hour would further increase the fluid overload and worsen the pulmonary edema. Pulmonary edema is due to an increased blood volume in the lungs. This blood volume causes an increased hydrostatic pressure, which forces fluid from the pulmonary capillaries into the interstitial space and alveoli. The fluid in the alveoli blocks the air exchange, causing impaired gas exchange. The priority treatment for these patients is to improve their gas exchange and decrease volume overload. Dobutamine is a positive inotrope, which helps the heart pump more effectively, reducing the amount of blood pooling in the lungs. Morphine helps decrease venous pressure, which helps decrease the pressure in the lungs and the movement of fluid into the lungs, relieving dyspnea. Furosemide is a diuretic and helps remove some of the extra fluid from the lungs.

113. B: Ascites (fluid buildup in the abdomen) puts pressure on the diaphragm, resulting in difficulty breathing and dyspnea. Paracentesis (surgical puncture of the abdominal cavity to aspirate fluid) is done to remove fluid from the abdominal cavity and thus reduce pressure on the diaphragm in order to relieve the dyspnea. Pruritus, jaundice, and peripheral neuropathy are signs of cirrhosis that aren't relieved or treated by paracentesis.

114. A: An NG tube is no longer routinely inserted to treat pancreatitis, but if the client has protracted vomiting, the NG tube is inserted to drain fluids and gas and relieve vomiting. An NG tube doesn't prevent spasms at the sphincter of Oddi (a valve in the duodenum that controls the flow of digestive enzymes) or prevent air from forming in the small and large intestine. The

common bile duct connects to the pancreas and the gall bladder, and a T tube rather than an NG tube would be used to collect bile drainage from the common bile duct.

115. A: Before starting a feeding, it's essential to ensure that the tube is in the proper location. Aspirating for stomach contents confirms correct placement. While initial feedings should be given slowly, giving the feeding without confirming proper placement puts the client at risk for aspiration. Clamping the tube provides no information about tube placement. If an X-ray is ordered, it should be done immediately, not in 24 hours.

116. A: Diarrhea due to an acute episode of ulcerative colitis leads to fluid and electrolyte losses, so fluid and sodium replacement is necessary. There is no need to restrict foods high in potassium, but potassium may need to be replaced. If the client is taking steroid medications, the nurse should monitor his glucose levels, but this isn't the highest priority. Noting changes in stool consistency is important, but fluid replacement takes priority.

117. A: Syndrome of inappropriate antidiuretic hormone (SIADH) results in an abnormally high release of antidiuretic hormone, which causes water retention as serum sodium levels fall, leading to edema and weight gain. Because of fluid retention, urine output is low. Fluid is restricted to prevent fluid overload rather than replaced. As the urine becomes more concentrated, the specific gravity increases. Other symptoms include nausea, vomiting, seizures, altered mentation, and coma. SIADH is most common with diseases of the hypothalamus but can also occur with heart failure, Guillain-Barré syndrome, meningitis, encephalitis, head trauma, or brain tumors. It may also be triggered by medications.

118. D: Serum theophylline levels are therapeutic when they fall between 10 to 20 μg/mL. A serum theophylline level of 25 μg/ml is in the toxic range and can lead to severe adverse reactions, which may be life threatening. The nurse should withhold the next dose of theophylline and notify the physician immediately. A theophylline level of 8 μg/ml is below the therapeutic range; the physician should be notified, but this level doesn't require immediate nursing action. Theophylline levels of 12 μg/ml and 20 μg/ml are within the therapeutic range.

119. C: The normal value for serum amylase is 30 to 100 IU/L, so a level of 306 IU/L is indicative of pancreatitis. Pancreatitis involves activation of pancreatic enzymes, such as amylase and lipase. Therefore, serum amylase is often at least twice the normal level and lipase levels can be 5 times the normal level in a client with acute pancreatitis. Serum creatinine level (normal value 0.5 to 1.2 mg/dL) is elevated with kidney dysfunction. Injury or disease of the liver causes elevated ALT level (normal value 7 to 40 IU/L). Troponin T level (normal value <0.2 μg/L) is elevated with heart damage, such as a myocardial infarction.

120. C: Semi-Fowler's position, or sitting at about 45 degrees, facilitates lung expansion. The dorsal recumbent (supine) position doesn't ease the work of breathing. The lithotomy (legs up in stirrups) position is normally used for gynecologic examination but might worsen dyspnea. Sims' position is a lateral position with the top leg flexed toward the chest. This position inhibits lung expansion.

121. B: With a bowel obstruction, abdominal distention occurs. Measuring abdominal girth provides quantitative information about increases or decreases in the amount of distention. Monitoring daily weights provides information about fluid status. An increase in daily weight usually indicates fluid retention. Measuring intake and output provides no information about abdominal distention or the obstruction although it is to monitor output. A client with a bowel obstruction will have a nothing-by-mouth order.

122. A: Placing the client in high Fowler's position, such as in a chair, uses gravity to reduce the risk of aspiration. Solids and liquids shouldn't be offered together because when they're in the mouth together, the liquids can cause the solids to be swallowed before they're properly chewed. However, water or other fluid should be sipped after swallowing to clear the throat. Thin liquids should be thickened. Food should be placed on the unaffected side to prevent it from being trapped in the cheek on the affected side. Using smaller utensils to limit bite size and doing muscle-strengthening exercises may reduce dysphagia.

123. D: Constrictive clothing, especially around the client's neck, can interfere with oxygenation, so it should be loosened. One should never force anything such as a padded tongue blade into the mouth because it could break teeth or induce vomiting. A client who is having seizures should not be restrained, as it can cause soft-tissue injury and musculoskeletal damage. Instead, any dangerous objects should be removed from around the client. Because a supine position increases the risk of aspiration, the client should be helped into a side-lying position.

124. A: After the client undergoes a myelogram (a radiograph of the spinal cord) with a water-based dye, the client should be encouraged to drink liberal amounts of fluid to rehydrate and replace cerebrospinal fluid. Blood glucose level monitoring isn't essential. The client should be positioned with the head of the bed elevated to pool the dye at the lower end of the spinal canal to reduce irritation of the meninges. Bathroom privileges are granted, but unnecessary turning isn't advised for the first few hours.

125. B: Cerebrospinal fluid (CSF) has high glucose content and would test positive for glucose. However, this test is not always accurate if the client has diabetes or a viral infection, so results should be verified by a beta-2 transferrin test. Testing the pH and the specific gravity of the drainage wouldn't specifically identify CSF. Brown staining isn't typical of CSF although the discharge may contain blood at times. Nasal leakage of CSF may occur as the result of trauma, surgery, or destructive tumors that cause fistula formation between the dura and base of the skull, discharging the fluid through the nose. This puts the client at risk of developing an infection as bacteria ascend into the intracranial space.